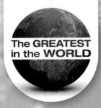
The GREATEST in the WORLD

illustrated by
Peter Bellingham

Beth Cooper

The Greatest

Breastfeeding

Tips in the World

A 'The Greatest in the World' book

www.thegreatestintheworld.com

Illustrations:
Peter Bellingham

Typesetting:
BR Typesetting

Cover images:
© Sherene Hustler, Inner Eye Photography
© Pavel Losevsky, © Valentin Mosichev; © Tomasz Trojanowski
courtesy of www.fotolia.com

Copy editor:
Bronwyn Robertson
www.theartsva.com

Series creator/editor:
Steve Brookes

Published in 2008 by
The Greatest in the World Ltd, PO Box 3182,
Stratford-upon-Avon, Warwickshire CV37 7XW

Text copyright © 2008 – Beth Cooper
Illustrations copyright © 2008 – The Greatest in the World Ltd.

A CIP catalogue record for this book is available from the British Library
ISBN 978-1-905151-34-9

Printed and bound in China by 1010 Printing International Ltd.

For Samara and Marc

And to my parents,
who taught me how to fly.

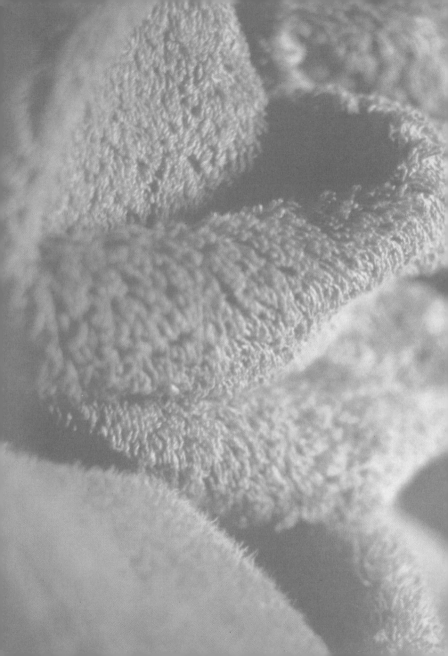

Contents

Foreword by Dr Nan Jolly

Breastfeeding, believe it or not, is not about the milk. It's more than just about that, because mothers' milk is more awesome, the more you find out about it. For that matter, sex is not just about the sperm either. Breastfeeding is an intimate physical relationship, just as sex is, and maybe we learn to have good sex by starting our lives breastfeeding.

The mother-infant relationship is the very first one we all have, and it's the prototype for all our relationships, for the rest of our lives. Breastfeeding makes a huge difference to those relationships. I think this is part of Mother Nature's plan – the reason why it looks so beautiful and feels so good.

It's comforting to know that we're designed to do this lovely, wise and fascinating thing, and if we just relax, follow our instincts and stop interfering, it'll work easily. Of course, this isn't as easy as it sounds, and supportive people around us help it to happen.

Breastfeeding is very simple really – it's a baby suckling on its mother's breasts. But 'simple' doesn't necessarily mean 'easy'. In today's industrialised and consumer-driven societies, there are plenty of mothers who will confirm that it isn't always as effortless as it looks; there are many pitfalls in the way of success and these, in fact, sometimes feel like systematic sabotage!

When I had my first baby, I expected to breastfeed and was devastated when I ended up bottle feeding; as a doctor, I had thought it came naturally. I learned the hard way that it helps enormously to be prepared with accurate information and practical support. It's a learned art after all and takes time and effort—even some pain—but is well worth learning. After I'd got good information and a strong support group, breastfeeding my second baby was one of the most fulfilling and seminal experiences of my life.

We know these days that a mother needs useful information, encouragement, and support to succeed. Beth's succinct and funny book provides the 21st century mother with the facts she needs; all she has to do now is set up a support group around her, just as Beth advises.

The beginning is the hardest part. So, get help if it doesn't go smoothly, hang in there – and don't forget to enjoy it.

Dr Nan Jolly

Dr Nan Jolly, MB BCh IBCLC LLLL

A few words from Beth ...

I became passionate about breastfeeding quite by accident. While pregnant with my daughter, I was more interested in morning sickness and maternity wear than the art of milk-making! To me, lactation was simply a biological process sandwiched between conception and motherhood. I had no idea that nursing a child was such a momentous miracle of nature.

My newborn's first brush with the breast was a comedy of errors. Neither of us knew what we were doing – and well-meaning nurses and doctors seemed hardly more clued up than we were. Ironically, it was probably my ignorance of the whole process that cemented my success. I didn't know at the time that breast was best – I just knew it was the natural aftermath, as it were, of giving birth. This meant I was blissfully naïve about formula feeding too; it never occurred to me to give Samara a bottle!

Modern society has made great strides in medicine, not least of all in the fields of reproductive health, pregnancy, and birth. Unfortunately, this has also caused interference in some natural human practices, such as breastfeeding. For years, Western mothers were encouraged to nurse their babies on a fixed schedule and to swap to formula milks at the slightest whiff of trouble. Thanks to enlightened experts and savvy parents, these outdated policies are changing.

Being a journalist, I'm instinctively curious and as a mum, fiercely protective of my child's well-being. When I started researching breastfeeding in-depth and discovered a wealth of information about the power of human milk, I was sold. More than two years later, I'm still nursing – and still loving it.

I'm not a lactation consultant or medical professional. I wrote this book because mums-to-be deserve a helping hand with producing the world's most phenomenal foodstuff. In the words of playwright, author and mum of two Karen Jeynes:

"Try it. Just try it. It might seem weird to you, your friends might tell you not to bother, but once you've got baby latched, the bond between the two of you is unbreakable, and you feel like a wonderwoman. Sometimes you also feel a little like a cow, but mostly – you feel like a wonderwoman".

Love

Beth x

A newborn baby has only three demands. They are warmth in the arms of its mother, food from her breasts, and security in the knowledge of her presence. Breastfeeding satisfies all three.

Grantly Dick-Read

Mum's marvellous milk bar!

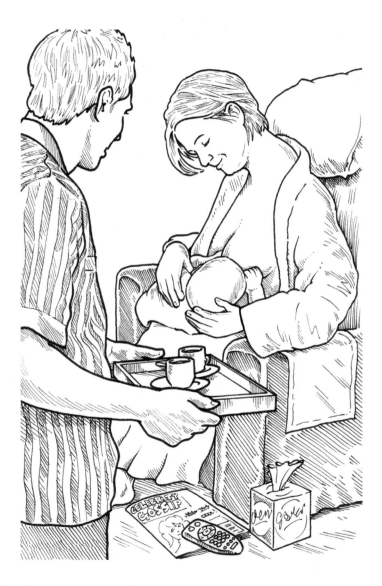

chapter 1
Mum's marvellous milk bar!

Birds do it, boobs do it

Everybody knows that breast is best, but getting to grips with a new baby and leaking mammary glands feels like rocket science in the early weeks. While breastfeeding is the most natural form of nutrition, it's a marvellously messy process of trial and error. You may leak, you may cry and you may toy with throwing in the towel. Don't, if you can help it. Midwives, health visitors, your mum, and the internet have loads of useful advice. Expect the unexpected and remember that it takes time to master the most important skill in the world.

Quick tip

OF NURSES AND NIPPLES

Did you know that the word 'nurse' historically meant 'to breastfeed'? Like these caring professionals, you need to be patiently dedicated to the task at hand to succeed. Today's fast-paced society demands quick-fix solutions, but your role in the early days is simple – nestle down with baby at the breast and get to know each other. It takes time and effort, so settle in for a breast fest and don't rush.

NANNY NATURE

Mother's milk is the perfect food. It contains all the necessary nutrients to build a bonny baby and what's more, it comes pre-packaged and at just the right temperature! The World Health Organisation (WHO) advises exclusive breastfeeding for the first six months of life. Those magical mammaries will help your baby reach her IQ potential, protect against illnesses, and promote overall health.

Liquid diet

Introducing a smorgasbord of solids before six months of age won't do your baby any favours. Nothing but mother's milk for the first several months of life is the ideal meal plan. Unless advised otherwise by your GP or paediatrician for specific health reasons, it's best to delay starting solid food until the second half of your baby's first year. Why, you ask?

- The risk of food allergies lessens.
- The risk of obesity decreases.
- Your baby is better able to fight off diseases.
- She'll handle solid food much better from six months onwards.

The magic of milk-making

Eye-poppingly gorgeous they may be in a lacy push-up bra, breasts are really more biology than beauty. When you realise just how complex and sophisticated these awesome appendages are, you'll have oodles more respect for the job they're designed to do. Many women roll their eyes in horror at the thought of leaking nipples and granny-strap brassieres, but know this – lactation makes science sexy. And no matter what your partner or his mates may say, everybody loves a breastfeeding babe!

Imagine a tree

There's a tree-like structure inside your breasts that makes and delivers milk. This lactation system consists of milk glands in grape-like clusters – these are your leaves. Milk moves down the 'branches'—or milk ducts—and then pools in wider ducts underneath the areola around your nipple. The ducts come together in the area under the areola—the 'tree trunk'—and feed milk into lots of openings in the nipple. When baby sucks, milk is released.

The science of sucking

There's amazing technology behind the traditional Madonna and child image – a mother with babe-in-arms at the breast. When your baby starts to suck, nerves in your nipple are stimulated and begin transmitting messages to the pituitary gland. This releases the hormone prolactin, which is in charge of ongoing milk production – a 24-hour job. So, every time you nurse your baby, you're ensuring that your little milk-making company keeps up the good work.

The big squeeze

As your baby continues sucking, the supercharged sensors in your nipple send another message to your pituitary gland – release oxytocin on the double! This important hormone contracts the elastic tissues around the milk glands, resulting in a generous supply of milk being liberally squirted into the sinuses and then out of the nipple. This milk ejection reflux— MER—causes milk to drip or spray everywhere, but of course, you don't see this if baby's mouth is fixed over your nipple and areola. If you ever express your milk by hand or pump, however, you might be rather alarmed at the uncontrolled jet stream that shoots forth. Many a mum has a giggly tale to tell about shooting milk fountains in the shower!

A two-course meal

When baby starts sucking, she initially receives a thirst-quenching, watery substance called foremilk. With more sucking, oxytocin shoots the thicker, fatty and protein-rich hindmilk into the milk ducts. That's why it's important to allow your baby to feed on one breast until satisfied, instead of timing feeds.

Love that love hormone

Oxytocin is much more than a stuffy old chemical – it hasn't been nicknamed 'the love hormone' for nothing! Each time oxytocin is released, it sends feel-good messages too and results in better bonding and attachment between mother and baby. As you nurse, you may feel a flood of happy, tingly, or downright dilly feelings. That's perfectly normal – it's mother nature's way of keeping you and your offspring joined at the hip (or rather, breast).

THE MORE THE MILKIER

Your breasts are, effectively, bottomless pits. No matter how much milk your baby demands, there'll always be enough to go around. This miraculous supply and demand system is quite simple – the more you nurse, the more milk you'll make. Frequently emptying your breasts of milk—either via baby or pumping—stimulates the body to make more milk. This fact makes mincemeat of the myth that you need to wait for breasts to fill up before feeding again.

Double delight

Mums of twins, triplets, or more can successfully breastfeed. Our bodies were designed to make as much milk as needed. Granted, it takes work and planning to juggle more than one baby at the boob, but biologically, it's absolutely possible if you really want to do it. A friend with twins simultaneously nursed her little boys for seven months and said she used this 'double duty' time to trim their nails and read a gossip rag or two.

It's helpful to know that even mums of adopted babies can produce milk. Isn't nature blooming marvellous? Fact is, there's plenty of information and support out there when you need it – you only need to ask. If nursing your own biological baby feels like hard going sometimes (in the middle of the night, particularly) consider all the thousands of women delivering nosh to a brace of hungry siblings, or their adopted angels. You're a VIP member of an amazing club.

> "While breastfeeding may not seem the right choice for every parent, it is the best choice for every baby."

Amy Spangler

Nutritious nosh

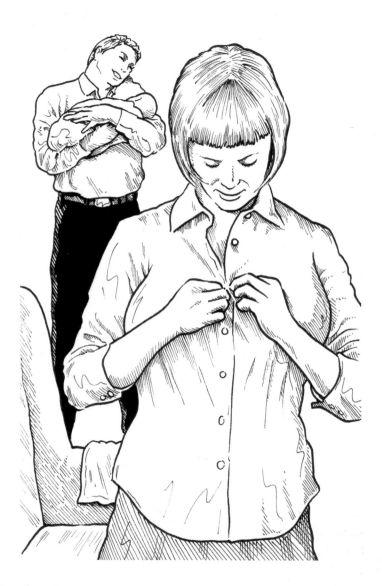

chapter 2
Nutritious nosh

Liquid gold

Scientists are clever chaps, but nobody has ever duplicated the complex mix of nutrients contained in a single drop of mother's milk. Vitamin-enriched formulas and fancy growing-up milks are second-rate substitutes, so bear this in mind when, bleary-eyed, you're faced with a hungry baby at midnight.

Colostrum

This sticky, sweet and nutrition-packed milk concentrate nourishes your baby in the first few days before your main supply comes in. It thins baby's excess mucus and helps rid its body of meconium, the thick, dark stool that lines its bowels while in the womb. Colostrum also contains a supercharged selection of immune-boosting antibodies and Vitamin K to prevent bleeding in baby – what a top-notch smoothie for a newborn!

Nature's vaccine

So powerful is colostrum, that you might think of it as your baby's first immunisation shot, without the hassle of needles and side effects! I love the fact that this wonder food was specifically designed to protect babies as they enter a brave, new world outside the womb. Colostrum is your wee one's big, burly bodyguard against nasty germs and foreign substances. If there's just one great reason to breastfeed, then this is it.

Disease-fighting duo

If you, your baby, or anybody around you is sick—or there's a nasty bug doing the rounds—crank up your breastfeeding sessions a notch. The miracle of milk is such that mum's body produces specific antibodies to any germ floating about your baby's system. These antibodies are automatically transported through breast milk to your baby, meaning she gets a double dose of Dr Healthy all in one go.

I'll never forget a rather horrible flu virus season when my daughter was just a few months old. Everybody—including me—was sniffling, snuffling and feeling generally under the weather. Samara, who was nursing every couple of hours around the clock, remained bright-eyed and bushy-tailed throughout, with nary a sneeze or cough. My friends were amazed and truth be told, so was I!

Bug-free babies

This might sound ridiculous, but you really mustn't stop nursing when you're sick. Logic tells you that you'll pass the infection to your baby, but this isn't so. She'll benefit from the antibodies produced against the bug, so stock up on tissues, take yourself and baby off to bed and let that marvellous milk do its job.

Obviously, you'll need to chat to your GP or health visitor first if you have to take medication that might be harmful to baby, but there are products on the market considered safe to take while breastfeeding. Always check first, though.

Clever clogs!

Some research suggests that breastfed babies have higher IQs. I'm not saying yay or nay either way, but at the very least, lactation consultants point out that breast milk does help babies to reach their IQ potential. Apparently, cholesterol and other types of fat contained in human milk support the growth of nerve tissue. When the going gets tough, it's rather useful to remind yourself that you're building your baby's brain every time you nurse — even though your own may be feeling rather foggy and dull.

Quick tip

PERFUMED POOP

One benefit of breastfeeding that seems to get precious little press coverage is the issue of poop. I'm not sure what your pet name is for stools, but a bowel movement by any other name usually smells the same. Or does it?

You'll soon discover, during digestion-related discussions with mummy mates, that the aroma of formula-fed poop is distinctly worse than breastfed nappy remains. In fact, breastfed babies' stools are actually sweet-smelling — until solids or formula are added to the diet. The grainy, yellowy, mustard consistency of digested breast milk is an odd, though welcome, sight. Your partner may well be cajoled into extra duties at the changing table as a result — yet another reason why breast is best.

"While breastfeeding my first baby,
I thought that I couldn't love anyone
more than her. I wanted to hold,
cuddle and feed her all day! But
I did feel that love again with my son
and now, 11 years later, I feel it again
with the latest addition to our family.
It's definitely a love that comes from
breastfeeding – oxytocin and bonding,
bonding and oxytocin over and over.
The bond that grew from feeding
my children is visible today. I would
recommend it to all."

Leana, mum to Mariechen, 15,
Manfred, 11 and Ilse, 1.

Feeder's digest

On the subject of stools and related matter, breastfeeding is kinder to the digestive system. Babies suffer fewer bouts of diarrhoea and gastro-intestinal infections and are less at risk of Crohn's disease or ulcerative colitis when they grow up. Premature babies who are breastfed avoid a scourge called necrotising enterocolitis. If you breastfeed exclusively for six months or longer, you'll also reduce the risk of food allergies.

Tip-top shape from head to toe!

By now, you're at least partly convinced that breast milk is rather fabulous. If there was any doubt, be awed and astounded by these quick facts:

- Fewer ear infections.
- Better visual acuity (acuteness and clearness of vision).
- Reduced need for orthodontics if breastfed for over a year and improved facial muscle development from suckling.
- Fewer and less severe infections of the upper respiratory tract and less chance of pneumonia, influenza and wheezing.
- Lower cholesterol and heart rates.
- Breast milk assists with maturing a baby's immune system, reduces the risk of diabetes and even childhood cancer.
- Constipation is rarely a problem in breastfed babies.
- Mummy's milk is also easier on the kidneys, as it contains less protein and salt.
- Less chance of reflux problems.

Sleep safe

You'll be relieved to know that, thanks to breastfeeding, the risk of Sudden Infant Death Syndrome (SIDS) is significantly reduced. How could milk and sleep be so closely related? Well, some theories suggest that babies who've died of SIDS slept too soundly and didn't wake up when they stopped breathing for a second or so. Babies often stop breathing for a moment during sleep; breast babies don't sleep as deeply and breathing problems are therefore likely to wake them up. The fact that breast milk guards against infection could also reduce the risk of SIDS.

Now, if you're considering, co-sleeping, speak to your GP first and follow these tips to the letter:

- Baby must sleep on her back and next to you, mum – no one else.
- Place a guardrail flush against the mattress – or have the bed against the wall or firm cot. Fill any gaps with a towel or rolled up baby blanket.
- The bed must be large enough.
- Ditch fluffy blankets, pillows and comforters – baby must also sleep under her own bedding.
- Don't bundle her up too warmly – body heat from mum, remember?
- Don't allow siblings or babysitters to sleep with her or leave her unattended on an adult bed.
- Don't fall asleep with baby on a bean bag, couch or waterbed.

Me, myself and I!

It's all very well to sacrifice time, energy and a pert pair of B cups for the greater good of baby, but what's in it for me, you may ask? Good question! Mums who breastfeed are richly rewarded for their efforts — and in the most surprising ways.

So, if benefits to baby have still not got you reaching for a nursing bra, take these gems to heart:

- **It's cheap!**
  Buying formula is pricey, while homemade milk costs only a wee bit extra in terms of extra food for hungry nursing mums.

- **It's healthy!**
  Breastfeeding reduces the risk of uterine, ovarian and breast cancer.

- **It's bone-friendly!**
  Women who don't breastfeed are four times more likely to develop osteoporosis than their breastfeeding counterparts — as well as hip fractures after menopause.

- **It's a feel-good factor!**
  Research suggests that breastfeeding mums have less postpartum anxiety and depression.

- **It's a fat-fighter!**
  Although much depends on your individual make-up, general studies show that breastfeeding mums tend to reach their pre-pregnancy weight more quickly.

> "A baby nursing at a mother's breast... is an undeniable affirmation of our rootedness in nature.

David Suzuki

Preparation is everything

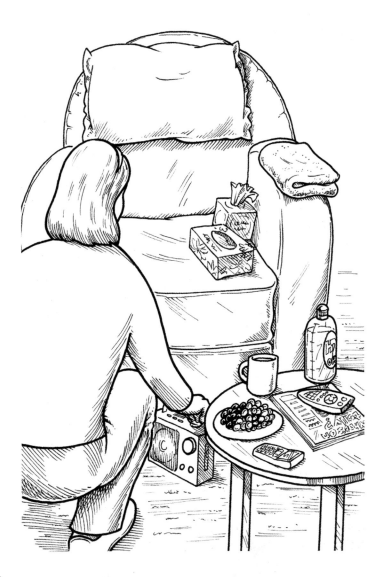

chapter 3
Preparation is everything

What comes naturally

When I was pregnant, the basics of breastfeeding were not
a priority. Morning sickness, tightening jeans and outlandish
cravings dominated my thoughts. Although I knew that
I wanted to breastfeed, the most information I ever gleaned
about it was a half-hour crash course at my antenatal class.

It's true that a few thousand years ago, new mums learned
on the job without the benefit of lactation consultants, fancy
books, or cooing midwives. But why eschew the benefits of
21st century living? Starting as soon as possible, get your head
and heart around breasts; you'll feel exceptionally wise and
holier-than-thou once baby is born. Preparation really is key
and there's plenty of help if you know where to find it.

The best of the best

There is a special group of women in the world who are
doing a great job spreading knowledge about breastfeeding.
International board certified lactation consultants (they'll have
the letters IBCLC after their names) are the gold standard of
support. Highly trained and tireless breastfeeding advocates,
they know far more than anybody else about the ins and outs
of breastfeeding. To find an IBCLC in your area, ask your health
visitor or contact La Leche League for more information. These
wonder women are particularly helpful when you are having
problems such as latching, engorgement and the like.

Nourish those nipples

You might have been told to squeeze, prod, poke and 'sun' your breasts in order to toughen them up for breastfeeding. This is nonsense. A little TLC for that gorgeous bosom might be helpful, but ignore the old wives' tales about scrubbing nipples with a toothbrush or burning them to a crisp in the midday sun!

During and after pregnancy, try these gentle tips to prepare your nipples for breastfeeding:

- Moisturise your breasts with a good quality cream or lotion containing Vitamin E. Try to use a product containing natural ingredients. If in doubt, always go organic!

- Massage a nipple cream into the nipples and areola twice a day. You can find these at the supermarket or pharmacy.

- I used a cream that did not have to be washed off prior to breastfeeding – this saves loads of time.

- My cream of choice during breastfeeding is Lansinoh – available at most shops and packs a healing punch! Just a tiny smear is all you need. Don't overdo it.

- Inverted nipples are only a problem if your baby cannot latch on and pull enough nipple and areola into the mouth. Draw out your nipples by wetting them with cold water to make them taut. Gently roll the nipple outwards with two fingers. Alternatively, ask your pharmacist for attachments that correct inverted nipples.

- At the end of the day, you really don't need to take your breasts off to aerobics class. That said, a bit of cream will make them look and feel nice – and that's super important when you're waddling about at six months plus.

Feeding station

I soon realised that feeding my baby took up most of my time – so why not be comfortable? Before your baby is born, set up a mum 'n baby area just for breastfeeding. One feeding often takes more than an hour and I found the following items very useful:

- Several pillows or cushions to support both you and baby.
- A blanket for cold feet (plus an extra one for baby).
- Two or three magazines or a favourite book.
- Bottled water or a flask of chamomile tea (you'll find you're very thirsty and a little peckish during feeds).
- A selection of healthy snacks such as raw, unsalted almonds, rice cakes, raisins, fruit, whole-wheat crackers spread with hummus or nut butter, etc.
- A packet of wet wipes or a towelling nappy to wipe up any spills.
- Mobile phone!
- In the early days, I even managed to write thank-you notes to everyone once baby was latched and eating.

A friend of mine really got into the swing of things – she caught up on e-mails and her daily journal by bringing her laptop computer along during feeds.

Where to nurse?

In the early days, you'll whip out mummy's milk wherever and whenever it's required. You're a mobile meal machine, so it's likely you'll have to set up a temporary feeding station in several different places.

When you're at home, however, it really is worth finding a quiet, peaceful spot for long nursing sessions. My brother lent me a lovely cushioned chair which I placed right next to the bed, within view of the window (to prevent cabin fever) and close enough to my bookshelf (to stave off boredom). Make an effort to create a cosy 'dining' space for you and baby – especially useful during lonely night feeds.

Getting to know you

A successful breastfeeding experience begins before birth. Experts tell me that most mums are hopelessly ill-prepared for lactation – and it doesn't help that health visitors and GPs don't always have the qualifications or depth of experience needed to guide you. Experience is the greatest teacher, but there are several ways to educate yourself. Start with a good support team:

- **Do your baby's father and grandmother(s) support your decision to breastfeed?** It's so easy to sabotage breastfeeding with questions like, "Are you sure you've got enough milk?" that it's crucial to have those closest to you on your wavelength – if they're not, you will need lots of extra determination to succeed.

- **Does your GP or midwife support your decision to breastfeed?** What is his or her opinion on nursing immediately after birth? You can often gauge a health professional's commitment to breastfeeding by simply chatting about it. Do they seem to know quite a bit about the benefits or are you brushed off with "Oh well, see how it goes and if it doesn't work, I'll recommend a great formula"?

- **Has your midwife or health visitor breastfed? Does she have children?** This might seem an insensitive topic to broach, but consider that your caregiver has a huge influence, especially during and after birth. Ask questions. If you have problems with latching, for example, what would she suggest? Nipping down to the shops for a formula tin or two? Or would she whip out a list of top-notch lactation consultants and offer to call them on the double?

Hello mum

Apart from your medical team, it's useful to find a close friend or relative who's been on the breastfeeding treadmill and lived to tell the tale. If your mum formula-fed all of you but still supports your nursing journey, that's great. It makes all the difference, though, to have someone nearby who can identify with cracked nipples and lumpy chests.

The world authority on breastfeeding just happens to be a bunch of mums in your neighbourhood, ready to share practical information as well as all the joys and fears, hiccups and happiness of breastfeeding. Join La Leche League a few months before your new arrival: you'll be clued up and have a support network all ready for afterwards. Contact details are in your phone directory and on the website (**www.lalecheleague.org** or **www.llli.org**).

Super sauerkraut

Don't just eat your greens during pregnancy and beyond – wear them. As odd as it sounds, fresh cabbage leaves are a cheap, effective way to treat lumpy, milk-clogged breasts and even prevent mastitis (breast infection). Buy a head of cabbage shortly before birth or at least within a day or two of baby's arrival.

When breasts are bumpy, sore or tender, cut a hole in the centre of a leaf, plunge it into just-boiled water, pat dry and tuck inside your bra while still warm. Repeating this with a new leaf every couple of hours works wonders. I found it both hilarious and uncannily effective! Another school of thought suggests a leaf straight out of the fridge onto a hot engorged breast.

"I didn't prepare at all. Didn't think about how the baby would be fed. 'Baby' was an abstract idea which had little to do with thinking and everything to do with a romantic idea. My preparation came down to one single, perfectly conjured image of myself in a rocking chair wearing a white dress, looking serene and apparently breastfeeding, since there were no bottles in the picture. I also had flowing blond hair, and lived on a farm. So the shock of having an actual real baby was, well, quite the most shocking thing that ever occurred to me. And that is no exaggeration. I was, for instance, outraged, OUTRAGED, by the idea that my baby would need to breastfeed so often and so long. I sort of imagined—if I'd given it any thought at all—that babies had breakfast, lunch and supper. Ha!"

Katya, mum to Rochelle, 7, and Mark, 5.

A thought on thirst

Since you need to drink plenty of fluid while breastfeeding, why not make an occasion of it by investing in a good, solid vacuum flask (for hot drinks) and a pretty, lidded jug (for cool liquids)? When settling down for a feeding session, I topped up my flask with safe herbal tea and filled my jug with homemade, sugar-free lemonade. Having plenty of fluids to hand saved time, kept me hydrated and, well, I felt as though I was on a picnic. Snacks matter too, but we'll discuss munchies later.

Mind over matter

When you have a moment, write down or think about why you want to breastfeed. Is it because the WHO says you should? Or your mum? Or because it just looks like fun? You also need to face your concerns about the process. Perhaps you're not comfortable with your breasts – or having a little mouth interfering with them! You might be worried that they'll stretch beyond recognition (rest assured, the stretching occurs in pregnancy, not because of breastfeeding). Don't just hope and pray that everything will fall into place. Talk to people, read relevant books, or write an essay about it in your journal. Sorting through your issues now is very important.

Be a bookworm

There are several excellent books available on breastfeeding. La Leche League's *The Womanly Art of Breastfeeding* is well worth a read and is available from any LLL branch. The large online bookstores also carry a slew of titles – try **www.amazon.com** for starters.

JOIN THE CLUB

If you're not attending antenatal classes or don't have a formal baby group, then why not find some pregnant mums and start your own? Some established baby groups might even be happy for you to join before baby arrives – very handy to watch and listen to new mums.

Milk that mouse!

I'm an internet junkie – whenever I want to find out something, I Google it. Whether or not you're keen on the World Wide Web, it's an exceptionally useful tool for new breastfeeding mums. Some of the following sites were lifesavers during rocky moments:

www.kellymom.com
– full of detailed information, resources and advice.

www.lalecheleague.org or www.llli.org.

www.breastfeeding.com
– support and information on breastfeeding, as well as handy troubleshooting tips.

www.sisterlilian.co.za
– an easy to navigate resource by highly experienced midwife, author, childcare and parenting expert, Sister Lilian Leistner.

www.askdrsears.com
– a progressive paediatrician, Dr William Sears has answers on virtually anything.

"It's a good idea to find your support person BEFORE the baby arrives, so that in those first few days, if there are any problems, they can be sorted out right from the start. A good beginning always makes breastfeeding easier. You can go along to La Leche League meetings before the baby comes. It helps to meet other breastfeeding mothers and watch them feeding their babies – and be able to ask questions."

Pat Törngren,
Childbirth & Family Life Educator.

Virtual sisterhood

If you're friendless, a hermit or live in the back of beyond, then joining an online parenting group is a must. I've made some lasting friendships with women all over the world – and have yet to meet any of them in the flesh! The best resource, in my opinion, is **www.babycentre.co.uk**. Membership is free, you're matched with a birth club and meet dozens of other mums as a result. There's a ton of advice on every possible topic, covering ages 0-3. The breastfeeding board is particularly helpful. Whether you're pregnant, have a newborn, or are a mum three times over, this is one of the most comprehensive and friendly cyber clubs in the world.

Motherhood can be a lonely business, no matter how near or dear your other breeding mates are. Faceless friends can do wonders for your self-esteem and peace of mind, since virtual parenting means you don't have to slap on any make-up or wait until a decent hour of the morning to chat to someone. What I love about internet baby groups is that you meet all sorts – and that heavyweight mum from Oz might just have the answer you're looking for in the wee hours. Weirdly, my membership of these parenting clubs has brought me tons of business too – networking across the planet is so much easier with other like-minded, financially savvy mums! We're all in the same boat and feel equally sorry for each other, not so?

It is only in the act of nursing that a woman realizes her motherhood in visible and tangible fashion; it is a joy of every moment.

Honore de Balzac

Ready, steady, flow – the early days

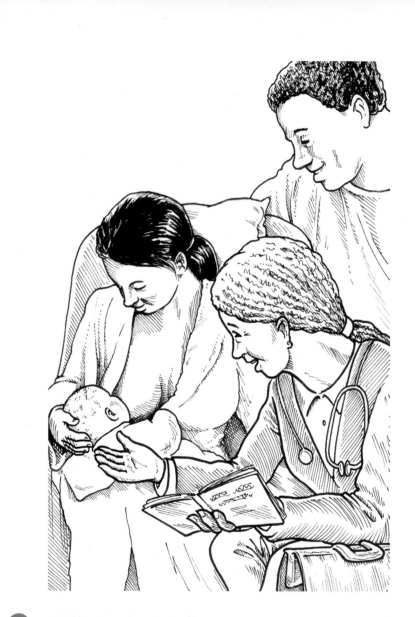

chapter 4

Ready, steady, flow
– the early days

Who is your rock?

Most women want to have a go at breastfeeding. What most women don't know, however, is that having a support team rooting for you is essential. I cannot stress this enough! Before and just after your baby's birth, let everyone know that you're committed to nursing your newborn. A patient, experienced female relative or midwife at your side works wonders, while having your partner playing slave to your snack wishes is a pleasant plus. This is your job now – ask for help if you need it.

From birth to breast

Nature's birth formula is simple: deliver the baby and then breastfeed. Modern mums are frequently separated from their babies or are encouraged to sleep apart from them following a hospital delivery. Try to feed your baby in the first hour or two of its life – this is when the rooting and sucking reflexes are strong and need to be practised. Doing this will get your breastfeeding career off to a flying start. Do everything you can to eliminate any separation from your baby; breastfeeding requires baby and breast to be attached – it can't be done at a distance. However, don't go thinking that all is lost if you are separated from your wee one! You might need a little extra help, but early separation is no reason to buy a bottle.

Know your rights

No matter where or how you give birth, you have a right to breastfeed and bond with your baby immediately afterwards. Many hospitals, and most birthing centres are now baby-friendly institutions which support the idea of keeping mum and baby close in those first few golden hours. When choosing where to give birth—and who's going to be present—bear in mind:

- It is possible to breastfeed and nestle with baby even after a caesarean section.

- The Apgar score (a test performed at one minute and again five minutes after birth) can be done while baby is on mum's skin. It's not necessary to place your baby on a separate table, as appears to be the norm in many hospitals.

- Speak to your caregiver about his or her opinions on the above. Enlisting the support of La Leche League or a lactation consultant will give your wishes more clout too.

- If baby must be separated from you—as often happens during a c-section—then she can be brought to you in the recovery room. I had to wait more than four hours before cuddling and breastfeeding my baby after a caesarean birth; what an anxious and tearful time that was.

- If your baby was premature or needs to be kept in an incubator for any reason, you can express your milk and feed your baby via a syringe or dropper. If this happens to you, call in a lactation consultant immediately – she'll show you exactly what to do and liaise with the hospital nurses. Any procedure that needs to be done can be done while baby is with mum or, failing that, dad.

Patience makes perfect

Getting it right takes time. Even if you've carefully studied graphic DVDs of nursing mums and practised surreptitiously with your childhood rag doll, real life has a way of forcing you to slow down and take things step by step. Accept that your first few attempts might be a comedy of errors and even once you're sorted, the whole experience can sometimes be rather energy-sapping and time-consuming.

Take your time

Once you're holding your newborn, breast at the ready, you may panic. This is quite normal. You will also feel rather tired, and that's when the thought of someone else taking over with a nice, warm bottle seems more tempting than an ice-cold beer in summer. By focusing on the fact that all you have to do is rest and learn to feed your baby, any feelings of guilt and anxiety should evaporate. Let someone else bring you meals, change nappies and top up your water jug. You're nurturing a future world leader, after all!

Quick tip

SOLID GOLD

In the first couple of days or so, your baby is drinking colostrum. From about day three, your mature milk comes in and even though it seems thinner (even blue-tinged) this does not mean that your milk is weak or inadequate. Nip those old wives' tales in the bud right now!

Stop the clock!

Your first few hours and days with baby are both precious and imperfect. You might have problems latching, fall asleep at inappropriate times, or feel terribly tearful and afraid to go on. This is precisely why it's important not to put your baby on a feeding schedule. By watching the clock and to ensure a bumper eating session at set intervals, you'll be heading for disaster. Why?

- Scheduling feeds interferes with your milk production.

- Babies' tummies are small and breast milk digests quickly – she may need to eat after an hour or after four hours, though usually more frequently than you'd think.

- By allowing a baby to eat at leisure, the biology of breastfeeding kicks in automatically and your body starts to make and supply just the right amount of milk. Crying is a hungry baby's last resort – a cry of desperation! The early sign of hunger is restlessness, followed by rooting and sucking hands.

- Your breasts won't take a lunch break simply because the nurse says it's not time for baby's 4pm feed yet. If milk isn't emptied regularly through frequent feeding on cue, you'll develop rocks on your chest. Engorgement isn't pretty and your long-term supply might be threatened.

- Babies know when they're full; allow her to nurse on one breast until she falls asleep, or for at least 10-15 minutes, and then offer the second one.

- A nappy change or nap might be in order after she's had enough from one breast. If so, always offer her the second breast afterwards and she might surprise you by launching into a one-hour marathon all over again.

- Don't record times and guesstimated amounts consumed at each feed. As you and your baby perfect your latching and nursing techniques, her nappies and general disposition will tell you that she's having more than enough nosh.

The beauty of basics

When in doubt, refer to the handy guide below – your golden tips for successful breastfeeding. Print them out, stick them on the fridge (and in your partner's briefcase) or leave them lying casually about where health professionals can't help but see them.

- **Latching.** The way your baby's mouth connects with your breast is of primary importance. Get this right and most other things fall into place.

- **Position.** You're going to be sitting on that chair for a rather long time. Being comfortable is crucial. Also, bear in mind that baby's body needs to be in the right position too, otherwise she'll strain at your nipple and struggle to extract any milk. Ouch.

- **Feeding on cue.** Timing feeds interferes with baby's nutrition and your milk production. Who wants lumpy, sore breasts and a screaming, starving baby? Work around your baby's internal clock, not the rigid, adult-friendly regimens drawn up by people who should know better.

- **Expert support**. Identify at least one person—a lactation consultant or experienced midwife—who can help you in the early days. Your GP is unlikely to know much about correct latching and neither is your partner, no matter how eager he may be to assist.

A womb with a view

You might have heard the term 'rooming in' bandied about during antenatal class or read about it in magazines. What this means is that you're allowed to keep baby in the ward with you, should you give birth in hospital. In days gone by—and in many hospitals still—babies are whipped into the nursery in order to give mum a rest. By all means take a break if you really need to – there's no reason to feel guilty about wanting some shut-eye. If you do feel up to it, however, having baby nestled up with you, skin-to-skin or at least cuddled on your chest, makes breastfeeding much easier, facilitates the bonding process and baby's health and development. If you are very sore, your partner or the nurses can change nappies, bath and take care of other necessities. But since baby will sleep almost all of the time between feedings, just lie back and let her smell you and feel your heartbeat. After all, she was curled up inside you for nine months and it's a big old world out here.

Latest studies reveal amazing facts about the needs of newborns:

- For optimal brain development, your little one needs to be in skin-to-skin contact with you around the clock.

- Stressed babies produce excess stress hormones, including cortisol. This is evident in several cases, including separation at birth, being left to cry alone, and when parents are unresponsive. A baby in this stressed state spends precious energy on surviving instead of growing and learning.

By rooming in with your wee one, you'll bond better, breastfeed better, and there's less chance of well-intentioned nurses sabotaging breastfeeding with supplements.

"I was knocked into reality and think I'm marvellously clever for being malleable enough to let the baby show me the way, instead of trying to make the baby fit the (idealistic) mental picture I'd had. It all worked out fine in the end. Breastfeeding is one of those things I don't imagine you can know what you want to know until you're right in the thick of it and have a million questions anyway. I mean, it would never, ever have occurred to me that there might be a moment when I wondered whether it was okay for my boob to be bigger than my baby's head. Or whether it was abnormal to inadvertently wake my husband by shooting a stream of milk in his face because of the midnight feed muddle in our bed when when my son and I were trying to negotiate the soccer balls on my chest together."

Karin, mum to Oliver, 7 and Julia, 4.

A bit about burping

At some point, you'll want to wind your baby. Some people find this a breeze while others—including me—just couldn't get it right. Many babies don't need to be burped, especially if they're carried around upright, like African babies lucky enough to be worn on mum's back. Try that for a peaceful baby and life! Thankfully, your baby will no longer need to be burped after three or four months.

The best time to wind baby is after she's finished feeding at one breast. This can be tricky if she's fallen asleep, but when I failed to do so, my baby screamed in pain after waking up. Winding seems to be important for some babies – too much air in the stomach is not only painful, but makes your baby feel more full than she really is.

There are several ways to work that wind:

- Pat baby's back while holding her upright over your shoulder.
- Walking around the room with her may bring up a lovely burp, or wear her upright in a baby carrier.
- Lie baby face down on your lap, with her head higher than her bottom. Pat her back.
- Nestle baby's back against your stomach and place your arm around her front, gently exerting pressure to release trapped air bubbles
- Massaging the stomach (baby's – not your own!) in a clockwise direction also works.

Some people are natural burpers – my partner could release our daughter's wind within seconds. I have yet to master the art of winding!

Fancy a snack?

Once you and baby have completed your first feeding session and she's snoring milkily, you might be horrified when she wakes up a few minutes later and asks for more. This doesn't mean that your milk is sour, insufficient, or not good enough! Few people realise that breastfed babies actually enjoy eating in 'courses'. Starters might take half an hour, followed by a little poop and nappy change, before the main course. After that, some babies even enjoy a little pudding. These mini top up feeds are quite normal. You'll find that after eating her way through several 'dishes', she'll settle down for a long, satisfied sleep. This is why scheduled feeds are archaic and pointless.

Gorgeous glutton!

Once breastfeeding is established, expect your newborn to nurse between 8 and 12 times over a 24-hour period. She may suckle for up to an hour or more, and this doesn't include breaks for nappy changes or winding! Feeding times vary, so simply settle in for the long haul.

Home sweet home

Although it might be the last thing on your mind, ensure that your home is a warm, clean, and well-stocked nest before you return to it. Assuming that you didn't have a home birth, you'll feel rather like an alien in your own space – after all, there's a tiny appendage on your hip now! The first thing you may want to do is just crawl into bed with baby – and that's a great idea. Take it easy and make sure there's someone to pamper you with a hot drink and sandwich.

Hello hermit!

The birth of a baby is an exceptionally exciting event. Everybody wants their turn to welcome this lovely new life. As much as you might enjoy visitors cooing and clucking over your cherubic newborn, it can get a bit much. Endless calls, knocks at the door, flowers and text messages become rather overwhelming. In some cultures, mothers are closeted in a quiet, private space with their new babies and attended only by close female relatives. So keep well-meaning visits and calls to a minimum.

- **Have someone play diplomatic security guard.** Allow your partner or mum to field calls and let people know when they can visit. A tactful, "Emily is resting this morning as her wound is still rather sore, but she'd love to see you at noon" is a good line to use.

- **Don't offer to make tea or rustle up a snack when people visit.** Your place is with babe-in-arms, no matter how much others want to cuddle her while you shuffle around the kitchen, clutching your war wounds and trying to remember where the fancy spoons are. If people don't offer to make tea—and there are those who do not—then just sit tight. If they're thirsty, they'll sort it out (and get you a fresh cuppa too).

- **Be a prima donna.** People are particularly eager to help new mums – you've just to ask nicely. Cast your eye about the house for chores and things that need doing. In your mind's eye, match a chore to a visitor and when that person arrives, exchange pleasantries, ooh and aah over the proffered gift and then say, "Would you be a dear—I just can't seem to get things straight what with baby feeding all day and night—and clear the cups in the sitting room? Sorry to rope you in, but you're part of my support team!".

- **Don't feel bad about leaving the room.** If your visitor's overstaying her welcome and you need to change a nappy, pick some fluff off your maternity tracksuit or go to the loo, then do what you need to do. A breezy, "I'm being so rude, but you know how it goes – please excuse me, have to 'x' or 'y' because of 'a' or 'b'." They'll soon head for the door or do something useful, like cook supper.

Breast blues

A hospital birth has its advantages — but leaving behind your Florence Nightingales for the lonely confines of home can be a daunting prospect. For new breastfeeding mums, it's particularly scary. However, the best way to deal with this is:

- Have handy the phone number for your midwife or lactation consultant and arrange beforehand for her to visit you a few hours after you return home. It's something to look forward to and she will remind you how to cope during the night.

- Don't expect to get out of your pyjamas or into a routine. Just plonk yourself wherever is comfortable, get takeaways and a nice cosy blanket and concentrate on breastfeeding. What happens between feeds is pretty standard. Nappies will change, faces are wiped and baby may cry for, apparently, no reason at all. If crying goes on and nothing you do seems to calm it, don't hesitate to call someone. Just having an experienced woman about works wonders. You will get through this. In fact, baby might sleep for hours on end, leaving you wondering what to do with yourself.

Sleep when baby sleeps

Caring for a baby is hard work. Breastfeeding a baby doubles that work load – your body is burning hundreds of calories during production and distribution of 'num nums' and you're waking every few hours to fill a growling tummy. Most mothers seem to blatantly ignore a biological miracle designed to help them cope – newborn babies sleep a lot.

- The average newborn may sleep 16-18 hours a day or more! What bliss.

- By one month, your baby will probably sleep for 12-16 hours every day.

- Although newborn babies usually wake every 2-4 hours around the clock to be fed, this pattern doesn't last forever. As she matures, the stretches between feeds will lengthen.

If you need to wake up, say, every 2 hours to nurse, then you won't be getting a solid 8 hours shut-eye. It makes sense to nab forty winks whenever you can. The problem is, most mums don't! We rush about writing thank-you notes, doing laundry or returning calls. You'll burn yourself out. Switch off your phone and ignore the doorbell – when baby sleeps, best you do too.

Try a tonic

Apart from any safe vitamins or supplements suggested by your GP, it might be worth investing in a tasty tonic – one that both increases your milk supply and keeps you peppy. I take Alfalfa, a sweet, syrupy concoction that tastes delicious and seems to work wonders all round. An elixir containing blackthorn berry might also strengthen and build stamina. Ask your pharmacist and always check with your GP before taking it.

Housework

People tell you to leave the dishes and ignore the muddy floor – but if you can't afford hired help, how on earth do you maintain a hygienic household? Seasoned mums offer the following sound advice:

- Only the kitchen, bathroom and bedroom need be hygienic.

- You won't have time to sort through baby gifts, so get a large box (or laundry basket, which looks prettier) and fill it up with goodies as you unwrap them.

- Store cards and sentimental odds and ends in a gift bag. People enjoy looking through them and together with the gift basket, these activities will keep visitors happy while you gaze into space.

- Paper cups and paper plates are not tacky. Get some fancy ones in gold (or choose pink, blue or yellow for a baby theme) and stack them up with serviettes in the kitchen. Add a few canisters of coffee, tea and sugar and guests can help themselves. Juice is also a cheaper, faster option.

- Ask three or four helpful mates to bake a couple of banana or date loaves – or bring a few packets of biscuits. Guests like to munch (and you've got paper plates – hurrah!).

- Takeaway meals are fine, but go for lots of salad and grilled chicken instead of greasy burgers. Baby and your tummy will thank you for it.

- Display your flowers and a bowl or two of fruit in the lounge – this detracts from the mess. Really.

Assemble your troops

The best time to have people around is shortly after you've fed baby, changed her nappy and settled her cosily in her Moses basket or on dad (or friend) in a sling. You'll probably have a good half-hour at least for a bath, a quick nap or a snack. To avoid freaking out your baby with foreign adult odours, give whoever's holding her one of your T-shirts or small blankets. Baby will smell you, even though you've shot off down the passage with nary a glance backwards. Other super-duper tips from mums-in-the-know include:

- Have someone sort through your gifts and make a list of people to thank – while you sleep. Better yet, get them to compose (and even send) emails or text messages on your behalf. There's no need to write laborious notes on pretty paper these days, unless you really want to.

- Ask a friend to defrost something from the fridge for supper and perhaps toss a salad (while you sleep or feed baby, of course).

- Practical visitors would be happy to swap tea for towels – get them to fold laundry while you wax lyrical about your birth story.

- When someone calls and says they'll be around at 3pm and asks if you need anything – well, yes of course you do! Make a list and keep it next to your phone. Have spare cash (coins and notes) handy to pay them back.

JOB DESCRIPTION: MILKING MAMA

Get your head (and heart) around the fact that your only job at present is to make milk. This eases up silly guilt about not doing your share of the housework, cooking, or idle chatting. If necessary, tell people you want to make a go of breastfeeding and are struggling a bit; ask everyone to pitch in because you fervently believe that breast is best and therefore simply cannot rustle up a vegan lasagne for your uncle's step-cousins at short notice, or even a salad for your family. Why do you think frozen dinners were invented?

Don't be a slave

Why am I repeating myself, you ask? Simply because women, bless us, have nurturing natures and despite all warnings, you're likely to be found in the kitchen most afternoons, cheerily calling, "one lump or two?"! Please – don't. Mothering is a mammoth task – pushing yourself affects your mood, baby's mood, and your milk supply. There is nothing wrong with sitting around all day in an old tracksuit, feeding baby and being handed endless cups of tea. I had a visitor who breezed in, holding a lemon meringue and then asked, once baby excitement had faded, when we were having tea. I had been home for three days and my Caesar scar was throbbing, yet I hobbled off like a happy hostess. A week later, another friend arrived with a cooked chicken and salad for supper, washed my dishes, painted my toenails, held baby while I popped to the loo and made me a flask of chamomile tea. Spot the difference!

Tears and torment

A friend once described breastfeeding as walking a tightrope blindfolded. Often, despite your best efforts, things just seem to go wrong and your first thought is that your milk is weak/bad/tastes awful/incompatible with babies. Promptly call in a lactation consultant if you experience the following and can't seem to sort it out:

- Baby is crying and seems frustrated.
- Baby cannot sleep.
- Your nipples are sore or your breasts are engorged.

Of course, you can also call your midwife or health visitor. Whenever you're worried, pick up the phone or bundle up baby and get to the local clinic or your GP. Taking action will make you feel better.

Quick tip

A PATTERN EMERGES

Accept that the first few weeks or even months are a mish-mash of mixed emotions, upside down days and nights and general mayhem. Something to look forward to is that once breastfeeding is established—at around three months—baby will settle neatly into a feeding pattern of her own. Even before that, you'll be able to plan a little outing or activity for the golden hour after a full feed. As you get to know your baby, life does get easier.

Phone a friend

Sharing your woes with a trusted mate has an amazing healing effect. I spent a lot of money on phone calls during the first month – and it was worth it. Having one faithful, patient friend on call for those wee hour chats makes all the difference. My office colleague Ursula was that friend – she checked in every day, was available when I needed to know what colour Samara's poop was supposed to be on day seven... that sort of thing.

Treat yourself

When all else fails, beautify yourself. This is one of the greatest tips ever – no matter how trivial it may sound! Get your nails done, have streaks put in your hair or go for a massage. You might even want to buy a pretty nursing bra and sexy, lacy underwear. A costly ego trip? Hardly. You're breastfeeding – spend money on yourself instead of formula!

Take a trip

Down memory lane, actually. Once you've had a baby, it's sometimes important to remember who you were and where you've come from. I got so caught up in being a mum that I lost track of myself a bit. Pedicures and fat slices of favourite cake won't cement your sense of self – but a bit of nostalgia will. Instead of madly sorting out your wee one's photos, cards and mementoes right now, root about for your own. See, there you are on your first day of school, all shiny-cheeked and rosily innocent! There's nothing like a bit of childhood past to put things in perspective. A cuppa with an old, pre-motherhood mate also does the trick. Try it.

When she first felt her son's groping mouth attach itself to her breast, a wave of sweet vibration thrilled deep inside and radiated to all parts of her body; it brought a great calm happiness, a great happy calm.

Milan Kunders

The low-down on latching

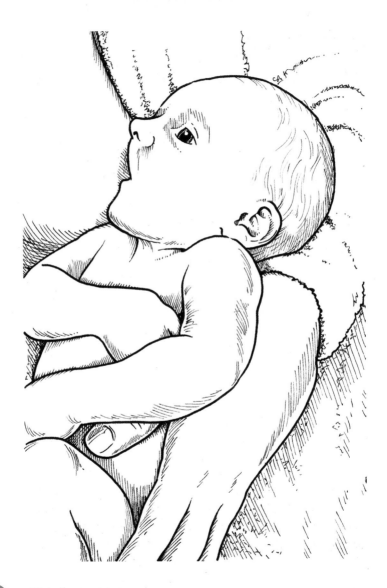

chapter 5
The low-down on latching

Here we go, baby!

Your newborn knows it wants milk, but usually needs a little help from mum at first. Connecting mouth to nipple correctly is the first step. Get comfortable, take your time and make absolutely sure that you get this bit right.

Quick tip

LOVE THAT LATCH

It bears repeating that latching baby the wrong way is one of the main reasons why mothers experience painful nipples, engorged breasts and plummeting confidence. The equation is simple: sort out the latch and most problems are sorted.

Baby steps

Strangely, very few people seem to understand the importance of learning to latch. We're so focused on getting going that the preliminary steps fly out of the window. Consider that successful breastfeeding begins before baby's had even a drop of milk. It's much like learning to drive – you need to get into the seat, learn where the gears and clutch are and feel comfortable in your seat before you turn the key. Keep that analogy in mind should you find yourself trying to rush things.

Relax and breathe

Before you begin—and this is probably the most difficult advice to follow when you're feeling all thumbs—relax! Become calm and centred by breathing in deeply through your nose, holding your breath for a second or two and then forcing out the air through your mouth. Try some of these top stress-beaters too:

- Exercise is a fabulous way to unwind and boost your mood. Of course, when you've just had a baby, you can't very well sprint around the block. Start by wiggling your toes and also get up and walk around as soon as possible after the birth. Clenching and unclenching your fists and rolling your shoulders counts as exercise too.

- Once home, light a candle and stare at it for a few minutes. Be sure you don't fall asleep and keep it well out of reach. Although baby can't even crawl yet, you may be a clumsy clod right now and are liable to send it flying with a nappy bag.

- Have a favourite snack or meal and better yet, get someone else to make it for you. I found that indulging in a childhood favourite around tea-time (mashed egg in a cup and toast soldiers) made me feel lovely and loved.

- Listen to music that you enjoy. It doesn't have to be classical, although ear-splitting heavy metal is unlikely to mellow you!

- Visualisation techniques are easy and they work. Close your eyes and picture a place where you have been really happy and relaxed – a favourite seaside resort from childhood or perhaps staring up at the clouds on an overcast day.

"Mums and babies learn to attach to each other with experience, and we can only provide tips. So the tips change with time when we notice some new aspect of attachment we missed previously. The rule is that however weird it looks, if it doesn't hurt mum and if baby is growing and happy, then it's fine. Only pay attention to latch if it hurts or baby isn't getting enough milk. And of course in the beginning, to prevent pain and poor growth".

Dr Nan Jolly, MB BCh, IBCLC, LLLL.

Get a grip

Here is the trendy mum's guide to successful latching. It might be worth having a copy of these tips handy – especially if you notice your midwife or partner making a hash job of latching first time around. As helpful and well-meaning as your supporters are, this is your baby and these are your nipples! Do what needs to be done to get the message across.

By the way, there's an excellent video available free on the internet – lactation consultants say it really helps to watch it. Visit **www.ameda.com/breastfeeding/started/latch_on.aspx**.

Now to the step-by-step guide:

- Wear a button-down top with your nursing bra. You'll be able to undress quickly and also see what you're doing!

- The rooting reflex causes baby to literally root around, looking for the nipple. Touch or tickle the lips and cheek at your breast to guide rooting.

- Your baby's bottom lip curls and the mouth opens wide. Cradle your baby's head and gently hold her mouth against the nipple.

- Gently push the chin down a little if the mouth isn't wide enough.

- Often, you'll be told to jam baby's head onto the breast, but any pressure may cause her to resist – and you'll see that as rejection! Many mums call this 'fighting me' or 'fighting at the breast'. It's usually better to hold her body via bottom and shoulders and use a finger to create a safety net for her head.

- When babies self-attach, they typically bob their heads and gradually home onto the nipple. If the chin lands up below the nipple, they will open wide and attach effectively often without any help at all.

- Most important – make sure the mouth is deeply attached, taking much more breast inside than you think possible! Imagine your nipple dangling freely at the back of baby's throat – it can't get quite that far, but the further it gets the less friction on the nipple, the less chance of any pain. If any areola is visible outside baby's mouth, there should be more to see under her nose than chin.

- Pain after the first few sucks generally means incorrect latching or the wrong position, so try again until it feels more comfortable.

- To de-latch baby, simply put your little finger in the corner of her mouth to break the suction.

- A good latch creates movement right up to baby's temples and your breast will be pulled deeper into the mouth with each suck.

- A bad latch results in baby's cheeks drawing inwards.

- You are likely to hear your baby swallowing, which is a sign that all is well. That said, I never really heard my baby swallow until she was about 18 months old! I panicked for a few weeks, but her chubby-cheeked weight gain and ready grin eased my doubts somewhat.

"It's all good and well to be told to latch properly, but sometimes between you and the babe, you just can't seem to get that nipple in properly. Then someone told me the following and it became a breeze: holding your baby in your arm ready to suck, take your breast in your hand with your thumb on top of your nipple and the rest of your hand below. Tilt your nipple upwards and point it at the baby's nose. Then wait. The baby usually has its mouth open BUT not always big enough. However, if you watch carefully, you'll see that every third or fourth or seventh yawp is bigger than all the others. That's the gap to take…when your baby's mouth is really big and wide. It's a bit like playing pin-ball…you have to await your moment and bang!"

Jesse, mum to Lily, 8, and Jemima, 3.

HOLLER FOR HELP

The first time baby's mouth connects with your nipple, it's best to get an experienced hand to guide the process. Although lactation consultants are the experts, your nurse or midwife has done this thousands of times, so consider letting her give you a hand.

Psychic poppets

Babies are tuned in. They're freakishly good at picking up your moods and respond to them accordingly. If baby senses that mum is in a spin, she'll fuss a lot more and latching turns into a marathon of moans. Remember that it can take a few days to really get this latching lark sorted. Your baby is not going to starve! Patience, support, and professional assistance, if necessary, will get you on the right road in no time.

Repeat yourself

While experience is the greatest teacher, it does help to have the latching technique burned into memory. Prepare by reading loads of magazine articles, websites, books, and pamphlets. Each time you read the same advice, over and over again, it'll start to stick. Of course, when faced with a real baby and a full breast, you might draw a blank. Not to worry – it's like riding a bicycle. You never forget after the first go, despite a few wobbles and false starts.

Look and learn

Try to watch a mum breastfeeding her baby. Attending La Leche League meetings is a good idea, but failing that, share your experience with other mums in hospital or, before the birth, be a nosy parker and ask a nursing friend or relative for an audience. She might even be willing to talk you through it.

Quick tip

I'M STARVING MUM!

A choice piece of advice is to anticipate when baby might want to eat. If she starts whimpering for milk, don't force her to wait until you've finished watching EastEnders. Not only is this very unfair to a tiny, helpless tot, but you'll find it incredibly difficult to get her latched while she's screaming blue murder.

Can she breathe?

If you have large breasts, you might be a tad concerned that baby will be squashed and unable to breathe. However, newborn babies' nostrils are flared, meaning she can breathe quite easily while drinking. If your luscious mammaries are very big and you're still convinced she'll suffocate then draw her body closer into yours – her head will extend a bit and her nose will be at an angle to the breast. Or, if you have to, with your fingers, gently hold your breast away from her nose. Usually, though, this is quite unnecessary.

Breastfeed – don't nipple feed!

Check that enough of the area surrounding the nipple—the darker areola—is in your baby's mouth. Many first time mums (and some midwives) tend to pop in the nipple and hope for the best. The milk isn't in the nipple – it's behind it!

Take a hike

If latching is just not working, try walking around with your baby, especially if she's very restless. The movement appears to relax jumpy babies and they often latch more easily in this position. Trying again with both of you in the bath may work.

Let-down reflex

When the hindmilk starts shooting through your ducts, you may feel a sharp pain under your armpit or in your breast. Some women feel a strange—but pleasant—tingly sensation in their breasts. This is the let-down reflex and indicates that the thicker, nutrient-dense hindmilk is on its way. Don't worry if you can't feel a let-down – this does not mean that you don't have enough milk.

Toss the watch

Clear your diary and just focus on the fact that you breastfeed first and do everything else second. Bearing in mind that nursing is your main activity now means you'll be less stressed and won't try to fit a thousand things into your day. Admit it, you were secretly hoping to bounce back to your former life. Why bother? It's the here and now that counts – and that means quality times with boobs 'n baby. What could matter more?

"Countless women have regained trust in their bodies through nursing their children, even if they weren't sure at first that they could do it. It is an act of female power, and I think of it as feminism in its purest form."

Christine Northrup

Position, position, ... position!

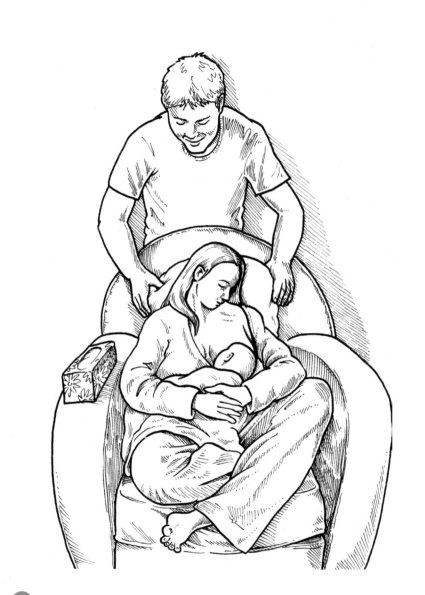

chapter 6
Position, position, ... position!

Jolly jail time

Lactation is a bit of a lark in that all the manuals, magazines and heavy duty classes seem to gloss over some of the really important bits – like the best way to sit on your bum after natural birth. Or how on earth nurses expect you to get up for a pee when you've just been floored by a caesarean. Breastfeeding positions are another area of mass confusion for new mums. You just pick up the baby and clutch her to your chest, right? Wrong. There's a whole technique involved in bringing baby and mum together for the long haul, so to speak. It's like wearing freshly laundered jeans – bit of a tight squeeze at first, but it gets easier with every wear!

Quick tip

FIND YOUR FAVOURITE

You'll be trapped in one position for quite a while during breastfeeding, so getting comfortable is essential. Both you and baby have to be just so in order to latch properly, sit happily for ages, and to ensure optimum nutrition (and lack of boredom for mum). Some mums love cradling their babies, others have been known to lie flat with baby on their tummies. Whatever works!

Hold it!

Remember my sage advice about setting up a feeding station? Try to create mini versions of this wherever you are, no matter the time. While your 'head office' at home may be equipped with several different books, pens, writing materials, mobile phone rechargers, a selection of blankets and even a television and remote control within reach, you'll need a couple of essentials to hand when nursing at the clinic, shopping centre, or even in the car:

- a towelling nappy or some sort of cloth for spills and burps.
- tissues or wet wipes for, well, just about any mishap.
- mobile phone (you have no idea how frustrating it is to hear that ring tone echo in the canyon of your handbag and be unable to reach it).
- a pillow, rolled up blanket or at the very least, a squashable bag for the small of your back, your arm, or your feet – aches, pains, tingles and pinched nerves are consequences of bad posture or lack of bodily support while nursing.

Snack attack

It goes without saying that a healthy drink, cereal bar, and a bunch of grapes are both delightful and necessary once you're entrenched in your breastfeeding pose. Trust me on this – you will suddenly become awfully hungry and thirsty when there's no cool jug of iced tea and bag of munchies within reaching distance. I had a particularly difficult morning when baby was just a month old – we were alone at home, she'd been battling to latch and once I'd finally got us sorted and settled on my comfy chair, I realised I'd forgotten to have lunch. She ate for

more than an hour while I cursed myself and silently starved!
Experienced mums will tell you that it's more than possible to
stand up with baby and walk to the kitchen, but in the early days,
a sore perineum or caesarean wounds make this very difficult.
Pre-planned nursing sessions are far kinder to your bits.

That's a wrap!

Swaddling your baby firmly in a blanket makes breastfeeding
a doddle, and positioning particularly easy. Baby loves the
snug, womb-like feeling and you have a better grip while trying
to find a comfortable spot. There are some well-researched
reasons why swaddling is super:

- Newborn babies become frightened—or woken easily—
  by their Moro or 'startle' reflex. This involuntary muscle
  movement is a response to a feeling of falling or loud
  noises. Swaddling prevents baby's arms from flailing about.

- Imagine being whipped from the womb into a big world where
  your limbs are all over the place and your snug home is no
  more. Swaddling eases the transition from mum's cosy cocoon.

- Over-stimulation is a common problem for newborns.
  So much to see, hear, touch, and do. Swaddling quickly
  calms down an infant suffering from sensory overload.

- The gentle pressure of a warm blanket might remind baby
  of the tight-fitting walls of your uterus before birth.

That said, some babies simply don't like being swaddled!
If yours is one of them, she might react to a feeling of being
trapped by becoming hysterical. There's no definitive rulebook
about swaddling – you do it if you can and don't worry about
it if you can't.

Swaddling basics

You'll want to get this right so that you bundle up baby in a flash before feeding time. It takes practice, but once you've mastered the ancient art, it's a breeze. Incidentally, my husband was far better at this than I was.

- A receiving blanket made of soft flannel is usually best.

- Avoid warm, heavy blankets.

- In hot weather, one of those 100% cotton cot sheets is lovely and cool.

- Lay your blanket on a flat surface (bed or changing table) and turn down one of the top corners (to about the size of your palm).

- Lie baby down on her back and gently place her head directly on the fold – about a third to half of her head should be beyond the edge of the fold/blanket.

- Tuck the corner at baby's left hand snugly over her body and underneath her right arm.

- Fold the bottom corner right up over her feet and body, below her chin. Don't cover your baby's face or neck.

- Now you have one corner left – pull it over baby's body and tuck it under her left side.

There are variations on this theme and your mum or mate might show you an easier version. This one worked for us.

Bear in mind that swaddling is best only until about two months old, as babies need to move around a lot more from that age. If you still want to do it beyond this age, then swaddle directly below her arms.

HOLDING FORTH

Once she's tucked up, you're stocked up, and both of you are sitting pretty, it's decision time — how are you going to fit together? There are a couple of basic positions but always, always remember there's no 'one size fits all' approach here! Play around, experiment and tweak until you find your Zone — that Zen-like position from which you're happy not to move for hours on end. Bliss.

Cradle hold

This is the traditional Madonna and Child image, though not everyone enjoys it. Sit in a chair with armrests, put your feet on a low stool or cushions and place a supportive pillow behind your back. Baby lies sloped down on your lap, at about a 45° angle to horizontal, facing you. Put your baby on a pillow so that your nipple is easily reached and you don't have to lean too far forward. Cradle 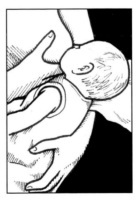 baby's head in the crook of your arm and gently tuck her lower arm under yours. Your other arm supports the back, so that you can hold baby against your breast, tummy to tummy.

Women who give birth vaginally can master this position fairly easily, but I found it too painful for my caesarean section wound.

Cross-cradle hold

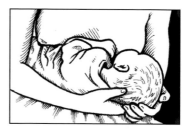

Related to the cradle position, but slightly different, here your baby's head isn't supported in the crook of your arm, but by your opposite hand and arm. Sounds confusing, but honestly, it isn't! Say you're feeding from your left breast; you would then use your right hand and arm to hold baby, turning her body so that her stomach and upper body are facing you directly. Placing your fingers and thumb behind her shoulders and just below her ears, you gently guide her lips to your breast to help her latch. Works well for babies who struggle to latch or those who are on the small side.

Frontal sitting hold

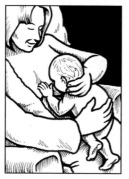

If your milk flows very strongly—you'll know because baby coughs and splutters or gulps—then try leaning back against a firm pillow in a chair, placing a cushion against your lower back and one at the neck for added support. Put baby on her tummy along your own, ensuring that her mouth is level with your breast and that she can latch on without straining. While this position doesn't work well for large-breasted women, it may be just the ticket for abundant milk-makers.

Football or rugby hold

One of my favourites. As odd as it looks, boy, is it comfortable! Here's how to do it:

- Baby lies tucked in under your arm, feet pointing towards the back of the chair.

- Your hand firmly holds her shoulders. The other hand is free to stroke her face or adjust pillows as necessary.

- It's best to put baby on a pillow to raise her to a comfortable height. I found that one pillow was sufficient when sitting up in bed, while two worked well when sitting on a chair.

- Since you will lean forward ever so slightly in this position, put a stool or cushions under your feet for support and also a firm pillow behind your back.

Caesarean mums and restless, jumpy babies benefit most from this position. It puts no pressure on your abdominal wound and for wound-up babies, the feeling of snug security under mum's arm is a natural calmative.

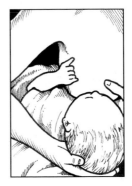

Twins also breastfeed easily in this position and it works particularly well for large-breasted women too.

Lying down

Oh, the joy of being able to doze comfortably while baby nurses! Mastering the art of breastfeeding horizontally was absolutely the best thing I ever did. It takes practice, but once you've got it sorted – sweet victory!

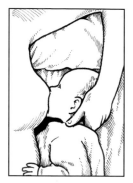

- Stack two pillows and lie with them above your lower shoulder, tucked into the hollow of your neck. Do NOT place your shoulder on the pillow.

- A large, firm pillow behind you and perhaps a cushion between the knees adds extra support.

- Have a rolled up blanket at the ready to place behind baby's back, to prevent her rolling over while feeding (remember, your arm gets rather tired – so why not let the blanket play the supporting role instead?).

- Lie baby facing you, head level with your breast.

- Do not place baby's head on the crook of your arm – she should ideally be tucked in the hollow between arm and chest and with her head flat on the bed.

- Neither of you must strain – mouth and nipple should be perfectly matched.

Tricks of the trade

Even if you were a pert 'n pretty A cup back in the day, chances are your milk-clogged mammaries will become rather huge and heavy in a very short time. If this poses problems during feeding, simply use a c-hold to support the offending boob. Place four fingers under your breast at about 9 o'clock and thumb on top at 3 o'clock. Yes, stop reading for just a moment and try it — quite simple. Got it? Right, now just ensure that your fingers below the nipple are more than 5cm (2") clear — even 10cm (4") if you can manage it. The thumb on top can be closer than 5cm (2"). Remember, baby wants milk, not your digits.

Quick tip

THE ASYMMETRIC LATCH
Lactation consultants stress that this is important to mention. There really needs to be more breast inside the mouth under the chin, than under the nose. It makes sense that the nipple has to be on top of the tongue, which occupies the middle of baby's mouth. Never fear! You'll see what they mean when you're actually doing it.

"When my son was three months old I went to a baby shower with lots of women with babies and kids. The other babies were being bottle fed and when it came Oliver's time to feed, I fed him there on the couch. It was my first major 'out' as a public breastfeeder and I was nervous and shy. The mother-in-law of the woman having the baby shower came over to me and said: "Wouldn't you be more comfortable in the bedroom?" and I don't know where the strength came from to be so bold but I retorted: "Would YOU be more comfortable if I was in the bedroom?". She was quick to say no and I stayed. Undeterred and utterly determined."

Karin, mum to Oliver, 7 and Julia, 4.

Lean on me

Newborn babies are helpless munchkins who need to be held firmly in position at all times. When preparing for a breastfeed, use your arms, hands, fingers, pillows, and blankets to place her in exactly the right spot. This is where swaddling helps too. And always remember to keep baby's body as close to yours as possible. Skin-to-skin or Velcro the baby to you.

Spice it up

Varying your breastfeeding positions might actually prevent clogged milk ducts and since your nipples are being pinched at different angles, depending on position, you may escape sore nipple syndrome too.

Quick tip

MULTI-TASKING

A note for mums of multiples – while the football hold is super-easy for you to master, there's another that might work well when the babies are bigger. The parallel or spoons hold simply means placing the babies on your lap, one head at each breast, bodies lying side by side.
You might hear people referring to it as the criss-cross position too.

> Mother's milk, time-tested for millions of years, is the best nutrient for babies because it is nature's perfect food.

Robert S Mendelsohn

You are what you eat

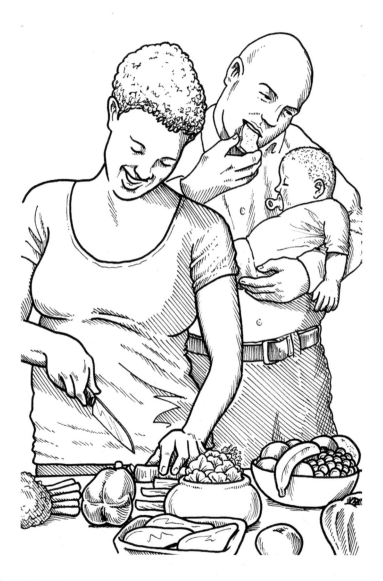

chapter 7
You are what you eat

Truth and lies!

You might have heard horror stories about having to give up dairy, wheat, curry, chocolate, and every other favourite snack while breastfeeding, but really, that's just not so. Following the same, healthy diet that you ate while pregnant should be fine. Of course, if you gorge on fried chicken and two litres of cola every day, your baby isn't getting the full benefit of a wholesome, varied diet. It's true that some babies react to milk and wheat - only time will tell if this is so. Naturopaths advise excluding dairy while breastfeeding and say that if baby suffers digestive disorders or allergies, then wheat is likely the culprit. But don't blame every fussy episode, tummy cramp, or sleep problem on your diet.

Quick tip

MENU MAKEOVERS

Look, even dieticians and nutritional experts have bad food days. The whole point about eating well is that you're obviously keen for baby to be well-nourished or you wouldn't be reading about breastfeeding in the first place. As your baby grows, she'll be eating what you eat and since she's part of the family, she's great motivation for improving the entire household's nutrition.

Stress test

More often that not, lack of confidence and sleep deprivation are major factors affecting breastfeeding. Before worrying about gremlins in your diet, always ask yourself if you are rested and relaxed. Dealing with fatigue and stress is important for milk production and a happy, hip mum. Consider this:

- When you're anxious about dealing with a newborn baby, she picks up on your feelings of inadequacy and helplessness.

- She may become stressed herself, displaying colic symptoms, rejecting your breast and generally appearing to be a poorly little soul.

- Worried and convinced you're an awful mother, you visit doctors and health visitors in an attempt to find the cause of your baby's distress.

- Often, when the reason can't be found, health professionals blame your diet – and bang goes breastfeeding!

Fatigue, lack of support and tension are major reasons why your relationship with baby—and breastfeeding—might suffer. Deal with underlying issues, focus on getting nursing right and problems almost always resolve themselves in a flash.

Baby weight blues

Another sore point for sexy mums involves how to lose those luscious love handles gained during pregnancy. If you're breastfeeding and battling baby weight, you might have all sorts of conflicting theories floating about:

- Will breastfeeding really speed up my weight loss?

- Don't I need to eat SO MUCH MORE since my body's an energy-chomping, milk production plant?
- I suppose I can't go on a diet now because I'm nursing. It's so unfair!
- I'm spending so much time learning to breastfeed – I don't have time to watch my weight!

Take a moment. No matter what people tell you, it's more than possible to get your life (and your tight jeans) back, even when you're breastfeeding! You can both eat and diet like a normal person – you just get to do things a wee bit differently. Making milk is not a prison sentence and it's just as healthy for you as it is for baby. It took you nine months to gain that extra weight – give yourself nine months (or more) to lose it. I'm still trying to get back into my jeans! Every woman is different and slimming down is not a race.

The bottom line

Write this out and stick it on the fridge. A diet rich in fresh fruits, vegetables, raw nuts and seeds (if no history of allergy), whole grains and good quality meat, fish and free range chicken is the best foundation for breastfeeding mums (and anyone else, really). All the minerals, vitamins and other important nutrients you need are available in a good quality, varied diet, together with suitable supplementation. Crash diets and processed foods will simply make you fat and unhealthy.

Madame Munch

Let's look at some basic food dos and don'ts during breastfeeding. It's true that some foods might negatively affect your baby and of course, you'd be a silly goose to continue eating caramel popcorn if it clearly gives you heartburn and mutates your munchkin into a mewling, spitting banshee!

If you've learned to relax and are aware that anxiety can upset your baby but are still convinced that something in your diet is contributing to nursing problems, then consider the following tips:

- Alcohol is best avoided, since it can creep into your breast milk. A little isn't likely to do any harm, but best chat to your GP or lactation consultant for expert advice.

- Onions, cabbage, and beans are common gas-producing foods. They're extremely healthy, though, and should only cause problems if you have a very toxic colon. Cut these out if you eat large amounts and seem to blow up like a whale. Luckily, baby is rarely affected by similar symptoms.

- Bananas, fresh unsalted nuts, and green vegetables provide magnesium. If your baby seems to suffer from cramps, discomfort or hiccups, eat more of these.

- Some babies are lactose intolerant – they can't adequately digest dairy produce. It's a myth that the best source of calcium is cow's milk. Vegetables, fruit, raw nuts, seeds, and even potatoes contain calcium. Do some research on this – you'll be pleasantly surprised.

- Good natural sources of iron are raisins, nuts, free range or organic eggs, legumes such as peas, avocados, and green vegetables. Iron supplements can cause your baby discomfort and raise the risk of tummy infections, so chat to your doctor about swapping to a 'food state' supplement or upping your natural intake of this important nutrient.

- Try to eat a varied diet. You might find the same old same sandwiches day in and day out are as boring and uncomfortable in the tummy for baby as they are for you.

- Wheat and dairy are common food allergens. Consider swapping to rye or gluten-free breads and slow down on the cheese spreads!

- Remember that even the most malnourished, impoverished women are able to breastfeed their babies. Stop fussing about food so much – be sensible, not stressed.

- Food is such a sensitive topic at the best of times – being overly fussy about it after birth will just make your hormonally-fuelled self feel that much worse. Simply do your best and don't beat yourself up with a cake fork if you succumb to your gluttonous personality every so often. For heaven's sake – thighs weren't built in a day and neither were health gurus.

The dishy diet

Counting calories and starving yourself senseless is not only harmful to your health – it just won't work! While breastfeeding—or at any other time, for that matter—a healthy, nutrient-packed diet full of natural, unprocessed foods is the way to go. Nursing mums are particularly prone to energy slumps and need an army of body-boosting vitamins, minerals, proteins other vital bits 'n bobs to keep going. Here's what you need to know:

- **Calcium** is always important. If you're lactose intolerant or simply can't stomach frozen yoghurt and mozzarella cheese, don't fret. There are plenty of alternative calcium sources and these are often easier to digest anyway. Green, leafy vegetables, raw nuts and seeds (almonds and sesame seeds are good), oats and fatty fish all contain super-sized portions of this mineral.

- **Protein** is found in meat, poultry, eggs, raw nuts and seeds, pulses, and dairy products. Choose free range or organic wherever possible.

- **Iron** is best sourced from natural foods, as supplements can wreak havoc with your body and lead to poor absorption of other vitamins. While red meat is considered the gold standard iron source, you'll also find it in raw fruit and vegetables (particularly deep orange or yellow types), preservative-free dried fruits such as raisins, green leafy vegetables and eggs. Some experts consider plant sources the best, since Vitamin C aids absorption and is found, together with iron, in fruits and vegetables.

- **Zinc** is found in high amounts in nuts and seeds.

- **Exercise** is as important as good food and supplements. Did you know that regular exercise actually regulates a bunch of hormones involved in the endocrine system? Also, natural sunlight provides your body with Vitamin D, which is vital for good calcium absorption. Expert advice is: soak up the sun for about 20-30 minutes daily (but avoid midday heat). Baby also needs some sunshine on her skin to provide the Vitamin D she needs.

Mutant meals

A sad fact of modern life is that food isn't the power-packed product it was, say, 50 years ago. Sourcing the best quality, most wholesome and unprocessed foods available is therefore way more important than fussing about calories and fancy menus. Ensuring that you consume nutrient-rich, unpolluted food as often as possible is the very best thing you can do for baby and you while breastfeeding.

- Some natural components of food are missing from our diets today. Blame petrochemical fertilisers, refined sugar, genetically engineered, and mass-produced foods and over-processing.

- Some studies have shown that the average modern orange might actually have zero Vitamin C! At the very least, there's been a 22% decrease in the mineral content of our fresh fruit and vegetables over the past 70 years or so.

Drink up

The best drink is water, without a doubt. However, always drink to thirst – don't drown yourself in litres of H_2O, since this does not make more milk, no matter how much your great-gran implores you to believe the old wives' tale! In fact, too much fluid makes you nauseous and can even suppress milk production. Too little doesn't reduce an oversupply either – it just constipates, causes headaches, and leads to dehydration. The expert rule of thumb? About 300ml (10fl.oz) per 10kg (22lbs) of body weight – and drink filtered, not tap, if possible.

So what do I eat – air?

It's easier than you think to be healthy – even if you have precious little time between nappy changes and feeds. When shopping or planning meals, keep these tips in mind:

- Buy organic fruit and vegetables if possible. Too expensive? Then peel the skins of non-organic produce or scrub them very well in vinegar water.

- Choose free range or organic meat, poultry and dairy. It's just not worth pumping your body full of hormones and other questionable nasties.

- Unprocessed versions of food are the best – brown rice (not white), raw honey, whole grain breads, fresh fruit and vegetables (not canned, freeze-dried or smothered in sauces).

- Avoid preservatives, chemicals and other weird food additives as much as possible. You'll find these in bottled sauces, tinned foods, commercial bread, some dried fruit, almost all processed food and, scarily, some children's convenience meals. Even commercial cheese contains preservatives! Learn to read labels — if you can't pronounce a scientific-sounding ingredient, don't buy the product! The E numbers are usually culprits.

- If you're a dairy queen, then go for unsweetened, live culture yoghurt and unprocessed cheeses such as cottage cheese, mozzarella, Parmesan and feta. Better still, choose goat's milk versions.

- Additives can filter down into your breast milk. If baby seems particularly upset and restless, check your diet carefully. It's really not rocket science if you just keep meals as simple as possible.

- Get mum, your partner or mate to whip up some homemade pasta sauce and perhaps some yummy bread. Freeze the lot and you'll have the beginnings of a great meal — just boil up pasta, defrost the sauce, toss in some cooked chicken, beans or tuna and make a side salad. See how simple—and safe—preservative-free meals can be?

Caffeine freak?

It's not difficult to make small changes if all you've lived on is fizzy drinks and café lattes until now. Start by adding good liquids to your diet, such as filtered water, 100% fruit juice (dilute half and half with water) and herbal teas (safe ones for breastfeeding, such as chamomile or red bush/rooibos). A great trick I learned from my very wise friend Heidi is to add a dash of fruit juice (apple is best) and dollop of honey to herbal tea — red bush is the best; this masks the bitter flavour and tastes just divine.

Count on carbs

Don't underestimate the importance of your daily bread. Well, bread isn't the healthiest option, granted, but remember that carbohydrates are a natural, energy-rich food group that keeps you on your toes. We tend to upset our bodies with refined versions of this superfood – cakes, pastries, bacon butties and the like. The best carbs are unrefined:

- Rolled oats (the ones you cook yourself or use in muesli).
- Baby potatoes in their skins.
- Whole grain or seed breads.
- Sweet potatoes.
- Brown rice.
- Sweetcorn on the cob.

It's what you eat with, and type of carb you choose that makes the difference. Eating a bowl of porridge with honey, yoghurt and a banana will keep you going longer than a chocolate muffin and a coffee, for example. Mixing carbs with proteins and fats will tend to make your meal low GI, therefore avoiding sugar imbalances.

Fabulous fat

"What?" you say, "There's nothing good about fat! How can there be?" Let's put this mischievous myth to bed right now. We all need good fats – without them, our health will suffer. I know this from bitter experience. A fat-free diet in my twenties left me with a damaged gall bladder, irritable bowel syndrome, a compromised immune system and, horrors, dry, pimple-prone skin and bad hair!

There are two types of fat – those that heal and those that harm you. The good guys are Omega 3 and 6, essential fatty acids (EFAs) that our bodies cannot produce and which must be sourced from food or supplements. EFAs control so many bodily processes and support our cardiovascular, reproductive, immune, and nervous systems. Even more exciting – they actually help you to control and lose weight!

- Omega 3 is the one most deficient in our modern diets. The best natural sources are flax seeds and flax seed oil, walnuts and brazil nuts, avocados, pumpkin, sesame and hemp seeds, dark green, leafy vegetables such as spinach, mustard greens, collards and kale, oily fish (salmon, mackerel, sardines, and anchovies), albacore tuna, cold-pressed and unrefined wheat germ, hemp seed oil, and eggs from chickens fed a good Omega 3 diet.

- Since we usually have more Omega 6 in our bodies than Omega 3, it's a good idea to up your intake of Omega 3.

- Cut back on bad fats from fatty meats, mayonnaise, margarines, fried and junk food, and increase your consumption of fatty fish, the Omega 3 vegetables and whichever other sources appeal to you

- Good quality Omega 3 supplements are also an option – either fish or plant-based sources are fine, but chat to your pharmacist or a nutritional counsellor about the best brands.

- Omega 3 makes kids smart! Children and babies who have a diet rich in this EFA are developmentally ahead. It also apparently helps in treating hyperactivity and related disorders.

Smart supplements

Since food production is a bit of a grey area these days, it makes sense to take a good supplement while breastfeeding. Be guided by your doctor, but also consider these excellent guidelines from nutritional scientist Heidi du Preez, who holds a Master's degree in Food Science and co-authored Naturally Nutritious (du Preez and Tilney, Aardvark Press 2005):

- Choose a whole food supplement – these are made of natural whole foods and food concentrates, without nasty fillers, binders or preservatives. Examples are kelp, chlorella, spirulina, barley grass, alfalfa, noni and wheat grass.
- Most commercial supplements contain synthetic, isolated nutrients that are not well absorbed by the body.
- Look for brands that are derived from whole foods or claim to be in a 'food state'.

The best of the best

For optimum nutrition, the following supplements are gold standard:

- Omega 3.
- Vitamin C – buy one that contains bioflavonoids. This means you'll absorb it better.
- Multi-vitamin and mineral – a whole food version!
- Probiotics – look for a brand containing Lactobacillus acidophilus and Bifidobacterium bifidum.
- A good quality calcium and magnesium supplement is also beneficial while breastfeeding.

"Many women decide to give nursing their babies a total miss when they hear that they have to cut out a whole variety of their favourite foods. Anxiety about colic is another deterrent and if baby seems to cramp frequently, a (mum) might well decide to change to formula feeding, convinced that her diet causes the problem. If baby sleeps poorly or is simply a fussy, restless little soul, the new (mum) will often suspect her own diet of causing the discomfort, through her milk. These views are reinforced, sometimes even caused, by doctors and clinic sisters, who often do not themselves fully understand a lactating (women's) dietary needs."

Sister Lilian, *Sister Lilian's Babycare Companion* (Human & Rousseau 2004).

Nibbly Nigella

It's not easy playing celebrity chef in the kitchen with a posseting baby flung over your shoulder. However, smart mums know that quick 'n easy can be just as nutritious as a slow-cooked, all-day casserole.

- **Double up.** Whoever's cooking should make a double, or even a triple, portion. Freeze what's left and enjoy it at the weekend.

- **Bake it.** All-in-one dishes that can be popped in the oven and left alone are heavenly. Again, you can freeze or refrigerate what you don't eat.

- **Drown it.** There are some good, wholesome bottled sauces available; choose ones without chemicals and which are packed with vegetables. One of my favourites is a roasted vegetable pasta sauce. I use it on everything – chicken, mince, veggies, rice and yes, even pasta! Toss in a handful of beans, a sprinkle of cheese or some tuna, and voilá – instant cuisine.

- **Stir it.** The Chinese stir-frying method is just brilliant. Buy pre-sliced chicken or beef strips if you're too lazy to chop. I add a dash of soya sauce, lemon juice and honey and that's fine for me. Add chopped veggies, spoon over pasta and drizzle with Parmesan cheese.

- **Relish it raw.** Health experts advise starting a cooked meal with something raw – crudités or a salad. A bit of lettuce, tomato and cucumber tossed with avocado, olives and even feta is a powerful appetiser, aids digestion, and fills you up.

Quality vs quantity

Believe me, you will get hungry while breastfeeding. It's true that we burn a lot of calories to make and deliver milk, but that's no reason to pig out and eat for two. It's the quality of the food that counts, not the double helpings of chocolate brownies. Nutritionists advise mums to eat to hunger and stop eating when they feel full. Focus on reading your appetite signals which are, most of time, thirst signals anyway! Is your tummy really growling or are you scratching around for an excuse to gobble a bowl of Cornish dairy ice cream? And when faced with a choice, make every effort to grab a fresh apple instead of grandma's apple strudel – most of the time, anyway!

Heavenly snacks

Most of the time, it's easier to eat on the run – or on the quiet, when baby is nestled at the breast. Snacks are therefore terribly important. It's all too easy to bury your nose in a bag of crisps, but cheap and nasty nibbles will take their toll eventually. Solid, nutritious choices include:

- Rice or corn cakes with avocado, hummus or tahini.
- Fresh or dried, preservative-free fruit.
- Halva or carob bars (raid your health food section for a delectable choice of goodies).
- Bran muffins.
- Raw, unsalted nuts.
- Crudités (baby carrots are particularly delish with a dip).
- Olives.
- Leftovers!

"Breastfeeding is the best thing you can do for your child and yourself! The first two weeks are not all moonlight and roses, but if you persevere, you make the best investment possible in your child's health and wellbeing."

Heidi du Preez, nutritional therapist, author and food scientist, mother of Christoph, now 4 and Caria, six weeks

Lady sandwich

I love slapping together two slices of bread – there never was an easier meal to be made in a rush. Choose good quality bread (wheat and yeast-free is probably the healthiest) followed by whole grain, preservative-free varieties. Sandwiches are a foolproof way to quickly combine a smörgåsbord of nutrients in one go. Some fabulous fillings include:

- Guacamole (avocado dip) and fresh coriander.
- Cream cheese and basil pesto, cucumber, tomato and sprouts.
- Hummus, rocket, sliced celery, avocado, fresh coriander and sliced olives.
- Finely chopped vegetables mixed with sour cream or cottage cheese, herbal salt and any other herbs or spices.
- Herb mayonnaise, chicken, celery and parsley.
- Sardines on rye bread topped with rocket leaves.
- Herb mayonnaise, spring onion, tomato, tuna and boiled egg.

Eat, drink and be merry

While the above eating plan is ideal, it's not written in stone and it's not a test – you can't fail at breastfeeding if you don't eat your green leaves or take supplements. Women with no access to basic nutritional information or quality food are still able to successfully breastfeed their babies. A nutrient-rich, junk-free menu is obviously the gold standard and it's always important to look after your body, however, don't stress if you can't achieve every food rule. Just relaxing, bonding with baby and getting enough sleep (when you can) is half the job done.

Thinking that baby formula is as good as breast milk is believing that thirty years of technology is superior to three million years of nature's evolution.

Christine Northrup

Troubleshooting

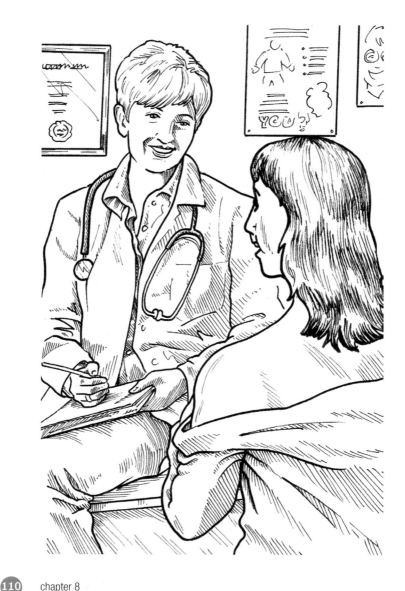

chapter 8
Troubleshooting

Breast blues

You will develop a freakishly close bond with your breasts now. Those mammary glands are alive, kicking and working overtime. As with any long journey, the road is bound to get bumpy—literally—at some point. Don't be alarmed when you hear the words 'engorgement' or 'mastitis' or 'bleeding nipples'. Your body is equipped to deal with these problems and so are you, as long as you respond swiftly. Bear in mind that most problems don't happen to most people!

Prevention is better than cure

I have a lumpy boobs story – it was akin to a B-grade horror flick. My alabaster C-cups morphed into blue-streaked double Ds with what looked like little grapes or cherries bulging under the skin. None of this would have fazed me in the least had I known what to expect – but this scenario was never covered in antenatal class. Had I known then what I know now, I'd have joined La Leche League or at least interrogated every nursing mum I knew before giving birth. Ordinary mums just don't have enough knowledge about breastfeeding anymore, and this is the main reason why things go wrong (and formula sales rocket). Plan of action? Arm yourself with knowledge and support. There are people out there who'll reassure you that cracked nipples and engorged mammaries are not the end of the world. Really.

Doctor do-little!

As kind and helpful as he may be, your GP simply doesn't know enough about the ins and outs of nursing to get you out of trouble – or prevent you meeting it in the first place. Generally, health professionals are not well-trained in breastfeeding matters. Even health visitors often rely on the same old wives' tales that we do. A lactation consultant, La Leche League leader or very experienced midwife, however, can spot a brewing problem well before it blows up in your bra. So don't panic – there are wise women dotted all over the place and they're just a phone or house call away.

Nightmarish nipples

Cracked, bleeding or tender nipples are a pain. This is such a delicate area, especially in the first few weeks. Some mums simply cannot bear the discomfort and give up breastfeeding within a few days or weeks. If you feel you can't go on, be proud that you gave it your best shot. But if you try these tips for dealing with nasty nipple glitches, you'll soon be back on track.

- Incorrect latching is almost always the culprit. If your nipples are inflamed, painful to touch, cracked or red, then you're not latching correctly.

- Practise your latching technique or contact La Leche League, a health visitor or a private lactation consultant for assistance. I cannot stress this enough – latching is important and well worth money spent on professional help.

- Lansinoh cream is a pure, natural wonder cure for painful, cracked or bleeding nipples. Massaging just a little into your nipples before and after feeds speeds up recovery.

- If you aren't able to find Lansinoh—though it is widely available—ask your pharmacist for a pure lanolin nipple cream that does not need to be washed off before feeds.

- Don't use soap.

- Ask your pharmacist or GP for a safe pain reliever if necessary.

- Sun clean, washed nipples for no more than a few minutes each day—avoid midday sun— and also leave off your bra for about ten minutes after each feed. Fresh air is a great healer.

- Gently massage breast milk into the affected area. This substance is a miracle healing cream too!

- Nipple shields sometimes do more harm than good. Be guided by your health visitor or doctor on this one, but generally, they tend to worsen the problem and don't treat the cause.

Quick tip

HELP! I'M DYING!

No, you're not – it's just a very sore nipple or a tight, taut football resting painfully on your chest. There are several common problems experienced by new breastfeeding mums – you may get away with just one, or be riddled with all of them at some point! Thankfully, there are cures for these nursing nasties and they tend to resolve quickly with the right treatment.

Chest rocks

For flat-chested women, the thought of tripling a cup size overnight is probably rather pleasant. In the cold light of day, though, engorged breasts are not kosher. A comic memory of early motherhood was drooping on the sofa while mum and husband manually rid my breasts of dozens of milky lumps. It wasn't funny at the time, but we enjoy telling the tale at dinner parties.

- Engorgement happens easily a couple of days after birth, when your main milk supply comes in.

- It's a simple case of what goes in, must go out. Not emptying your breasts often enough will result in excess milk build-up.

- Feed on cue—as often as you or baby like—and don't time feeds or nurse according to a schedule.

- Apart from feeding baby as often as possible, and allowing her to finish completely on each breast, you might want to empty the milk manually by hand massaging the blocked milk ducts. Massage gently, but firmly, towards the nipple. This will not make the problem worse.

- Alternate cold and warm compresses. This gets the milk flowing nicely.

- Cabbage leaves are traditional standbys. Use straight out of the fridge or plunge a leaf into just-boiled water, shake off excess liquid, cut a hole for your nipple and tuck inside your bra, changing a couple of hours later.

Thrush flush

So one morning you wake up with stabbing pains in your breasts. More often than not, you try to imagine them away – after all, strange sensations are nothing new on this marvellously messy journey. But those mystery jabs are often symptomatic of a thrush infection and this means prompt treatment for both you and baby. Once again, prevention is the best cure.

- Thrush—or a yeast infection—is irritating and easily passed between yourself and baby. Apart from very sore, tender nipples and shooting pains before, during or after feeding, there may be white patches inside your baby's cheeks.

- Thrush is caused by yeast growing out of control in our bodies. Moist, warm conditions are five-star luxury hotels to yeast. Milk is therefore the perfect getaway.

- Various things contribute to yeast overgrowth, including antibiotics, the contraceptive pill, cortisone, diabetes, very restrictive clothing, perfumes, a compromised immune system and simply being pregnant!

- Get to the GP for a diagnosis – both you and baby will be given treatment. Meanwhile, try eating live culture yoghurt containing lactobacillus acidophilus, ditch the lavender-scented bubble baths, wear comfortable cotton clothing, don't douche, and avoid antiobiotics.

- Don't stop breastfeeding.

The lump stops here

As if misbehaving nipples and weighty watermelons aren't enough, you might find yourself face-to-face with some oddly-shaped mounds and bumps one morning. Though sometimes sore and quite sensitive, masses on your breasts are usually harmless and more often than not, caused by blocked milk ducts.

- Milk ducts, like facial pores, do get blocked from time to time. To prevent this happening, frequent feeding on cue and hand or pump expressing between feeds to treat engorgement should nip any potential problems in the bud.

- Apply all the tips for engorgement, such as cabbage leaves and compresses. This too shall pass – really!

- Clear the diary for a few days over this period. When it happened to me on holiday, I shut the bedroom door, dunked my boobs in a bath of warm water and then spent hours lying with my baby, merrily encouraging her to nurse at will. Occasionally, close family members popped in with tea and biscuits. All were amused to see a wild woman, stripped to the waist, clutching warm facecloths to her chest and wringing out cabbage leaves. I laugh about this now. You will too.

- When all else fails, cry a lot and feel sorry for yourself. Expressing isn't just about lumps of clogged milk – it's about feelings too! Someone who's never breastfed or coped with helium balloons on his chest won't really understand. If there's nobody about to empathise, pop online to find a friend.

Going bump in the night

It's definitely not a blocked milk duct... so what is it?
There are lesser known bumpy bits that might cause you grief.
Since these aren't common, you probably won't find references
in your pretty preggy books or health visitor's manual!

- **Montgomery gland infections**. The ol' montgomeries are
  situated in the areolae (the area surrounding your nipples)
  and can flare up thanks to an infected cut or pressure.
  These are rather painful, but not serious. The best way to
  clear them up is to breastfeed frequently, regularly soak
  the infected area in warm water before nursing, and
  massage the lump gently.

- **Galactoceles** (what an odd name!) are nodules caused
  by blocked milk ducts. These usually don't occur until you
  start weaning. While there's no way to prevent them, per se,
  they either disappear on their own or can be aspirated by
  your GP.

- **Milk blisters**—'milk under the skin'—result from milk
  pooling beneath a thin layer of skin growing over a milk
  duct. You might notice a clear, yellow or white dot in the
  centre of the blister. This in itself will scare you witless, but
  home treatments sort the problem promptly. Try Epsom-salt
  or warm olive oil soaks and then a hot compress before
  nursing. The blister will probably burst naturally, but if it
  doesn't, you can very gently scrape away the skin with
  a clean fingernail between feeds. Your pharmacist or GP will
  advise on a healing cream for the blister area (but
  don't forget to wash it off before baby nurses).

Managing mastitis

This legendary infection tends to strike fear into the hearts of new mums — much like the "He Who Must Not Be Named" character in Harry Potter. However, mastitis—like Voldemort—is easily and speedily sorted with the right treatment.

- The symptoms you're looking at are wide-ranging. They include fatigue, fever, nausea, chill and a very shiny, red, hot and painful area on one of your breasts. In short, you will feel and look unwell.

- The minute you suspect mastitis, contact your GP. Antibiotics and bed rest may be prescribed.

- Mastitis is usually caused by torn, damaged skin around the nipples, blocked milk ducts or engorgement

- Lactation experts suggest that you continue nursing, starting always with the non-infected breast (painful, I know) until you feel a let-down reflex. Then switch to the infected side.

- Your GP will check to see if you have an abscess (a rare occurrence) and will drain it if necessary.

- If you DO have an abscess, get in contact with a lactation consultant immediately! They have much more in-depth knowledge about how to manage breastfeeding during this period. Your average health professional would probably tell you to stop nursing.

"I never realised that I had been given a huge dose of antibiotics when I had the C-section, and I didn't know you could get thrush in your breasts. I had no idea what the agonising stabbing pains were all about. It didn't help that I put the Lansinoh straight on the nipples without drying them first. I thought the pain must mean I was cracking, and that would help. Meantime it was thrush, and I was making it worse! As for 'just one dose of Fluconazole will put you right' (said one doctor), or just 'lots of live yoghurt' (said the other): Ha. Ha. Ha. Repeated multiple medications plus a heavy probiotic regimen plus a couple of months of special diet plus getting decent sleep again is what it took. No less."

Jean, 38, mum to Ben, 2.

Out and about

At some point—possibly just days after having baby—you'll want to leave the house. Why would such a routine event feature in a Troubleshooting chapter? Simple. You might be concerned that some people are likely to cause trouble for breastfeeding mums on the move. Breastfeeding should be a public non-event.

Quick tip

ATTITUDE IS EVERYTHING

You need to prepare mentally if you're feeling shy. Tell yourself that if people get upset by looking at something so normal and beautiful, then they are simply jealous (likely if women) or childish (male reactions). Alternatively, they have a deep-seated problem that needs therapy – and they should get a therapist or get over it. They could also just look somewhere else!

Slowly does it

The prospect of a public feeding might scare even the most Earth Motherish among us. The first step in conquering your concerns is accepting what a small minority might find unacceptable – you are a breastfeeding mum who will feed your baby wherever and whenever you wish. Once that's sorted in your head, all you need do is find a comfortable way of doing what comes naturally.

Managing mobile milk

Traditionally, we're advised to drape a nappy or receiving blanket over one shoulder, tuck baby underneath and voilá – a private nursing station. I suppose that works for some people, but it didn't for me. When outside, my blanket flapped in the wind, smacked me in the face and exposed a goodly amount of flesh. Inside was no better – my baby absolutely hated being hidden from view. The slightest hint of a cover up sent her spewing out my nipple in favour of a loud caterwaul.

Simply practise in front of a mirror first and always wear separates when you go out. There's nothing more annoying than fiddling with complicated clothes when a blouse or T-shirt would've made the job much easier.

Public feeding spots

These are the bane of breastfeeders everywhere. Okay, perhaps some shopping malls have pulled up their socks, but most of the time, I'm appalled by the standard of facilities offered to mums and babies. Still, scout around – where's the baby room in your local hangout and do you need a key to get in? If it's a dodgy-looking cell with an overflowing nappy bin and rather grubby, get hold of the manager immediately (that very day!) and lodge a complaint.

"Never be afraid to breastfeed in public. I went from being someone who would never even remove a sock in front of other people, to being a brazen breast barer in the space of nine months. You are feeding your baby, not breaching decency laws or disturbing the peace! Anyone who doesn't like it can look in the other direction – or get a life!"

Kelly Rose Bradford, mum to William, 4.

Toilet humour

Yes, there's something oddly funny about feeding your baby while performing ablutions – and many, many mums have done this. Not so funny is feeling pressurised to shut yourself away in a private space simply to nurse, or because the only chair anywhere is the toilet seat lid. Before feeding your baby in a public toilet, ask yourself: would you eat your lunch sandwich while sitting on the potty? Not likely.

Armed and experienced

Each time you venture out with your baby, you'll learn something new. The first few occasions might be hiccup-free and then again, they may not. But after some time, social occasions will be so much old hat and a breastfeeding breeze. I found that being terribly organised and prepared just made me feel better, even if nothing went according to plan. My personal recipe for success evolved thus :

- Feed your baby as much as is comfortable before you go out. The golden hour after a full feed is quite calm and heavenly.

- Don't wear a new, fiddly top or bra just to look pretty. Tried and trusted is better than gorgeous but hysterical.

- Have your nappy bag fully stocked and loaded with enough arsenal to cope with any disaster. An extra top, breast pads, little toys, a blanket or two, some Rescue Remedy drops, more nappies and changing accessories than you'll ever need and even a snack or two are handy. The food bit works wonders if you didn't have time to eat and are ravished by the time you head back to your car!

> When she first felt her son's groping mouth attach itself to her breast, a wave of sweet vibration thrilled deep inside and radiated to all parts of her body; it brought a great calm happiness, a great happy calm.

Milan Kunders

Weighty matters

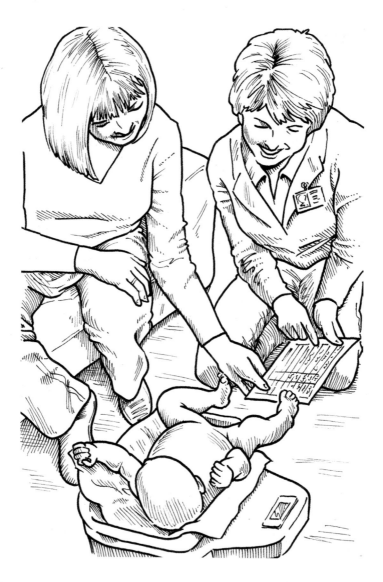

chapter 9
Weighty matters

Here we grow

It seems so easy to monitor baby's meal times when you're bottle-feeding. Wouldn't it be wonderful if our breasts were transparent and had measurement markings? But they don't – and the human race has got along just fine without complicated growth charts and metal scales. Using weight gain as the yardstick for whether or not you have enough milk—and if baby is getting enough—is fraught with misinformation and myth. Your milk-making ability is simply not determined by the number of grams little one has gained in a week. In this arena, science has failed breastfeeding mothers.

Testing tots

If you're advised to test-weigh your infant, run a mile. This outdated, error-riddled procedure can seriously scupper your breastfeeding plans. The process involves weighing your baby before a feed and then straight after she has nursed. The difference between her before and after weight is supposed to calculate how much milk she's drunk, and whether or not she needs supplementary formula feeds.

Problem is, babies don't want to drink to schedule and might have more or less during one particular feeding, depending on how they feel. After all, you don't drink or eat exactly the same amount at each sitting, do you?

Grappling with growth charts

I studiously memorised my baby's growth chart in the first few weeks. I knew exactly where to plot her growth, based on birth weight and could calculate in a flash how tall she was likely to be at age 4. But remember that growth charts aren't tests – you don't have to get your little one into the 100th percentile at all costs! And there's no free bag of nappies as first prize if you do. The chart is simply based on a statistical distribution of measurements in a group of babies. Remember half of the normal population is above, and half below average. Who wants to be average? Healthy people come in all shapes, heights and sizes – there are loads of other factors to consider. These are:

- Your and your partner's height and size? Are you a pint-sized poppet or a strapping Amazon? Siblings, grandparents and extended family all share the same genetic heritage too – so she might take after one of them, not so?

- Is baby gaining weight consistently, even if she's not shooting up the scales? Regular growth is far important than piling on the pounds.

- How about developmental milestones? Pretty much on target, give or take a few weeks (sometimes months)?

- A happy, active and wired-to-the-world baby who wets and soils nappies with gay abandon is doing just fine.

The real test

There are some solid clues that your baby is getting plenty of milk and that you're making plenty of it:

- About five to six wet or dirty nappies a day.
- Moist, sparkling eyes.
- Reaching milestones.
- Alert and energetic during awake periods.

Naturally, you will want to weigh your baby – but the above criteria are the main yardsticks you should use. Using weight as the sole indicator of your baby's health can cause stress, sleepless nights and in many cases, lack of confidence in your breastfeeding relationship.

Quick tip

SQUARE NIPPLE, ROUND HOLE

Many mums are unaware that standard growth charts are based on data from formula-fed babies who were not exclusively breastfed for the first six months – they started solids early. Also, breast babies tend to pick up weight really fast in the first couple of months or so and then slow down, while their formula-fed mates continue gaining steadily and generously. No wonder many doctors and health visitors give ignorant advice to nervous breastfeeding mums, suggesting supplementary feeds. The WHO has now revised these charts to better reflect breast babies' growth, but still, weight gain is absolutely not the crux of the matter.

THE WEIGH-IN

Now, if you do weigh your baby, always do it at the same time of day, in the same clothes or only a vest and either before or after a feed every time. The scales can be very misleading if you chop and change, resulting in unnecessary stress for a breastfeeding mom and mutterings about supplement feeds.

Wait a week

If baby is healthy and you're not overly concerned about her generally, then why weigh every few days? This is often too soon to accurately assess growth. At the very least, don't weigh more than once a week. For heaven's sake, you've got enough on your plate without a dreaded visit to the scales of doom!

Follow her lead

The commonsense rules of early feeding will influence baby's growth – don't nurse on schedule and always allow her to finish one breast before swapping sides. Some babies drink quickly, others take their time. Start feeding from the most full, taut breast.

Wet wisdom

If your baby's urine is very concentrated—strong-smelling and dark—there may be some concern that you might have too little milk at a particular point. Light-coloured and clear fluid is the sign of adequate hydration and nutrition – so conduct a quick inspection during nappy changes for peace of mind.

Super-sizing your supply

If you suspect that you need to make more milk, there are ways to get sorted without resorting to supplementary feeds.

- **Learn to latch and position properly.** Ensuring that milk is being transferred effectively from breast to baby is unbelievably important. Incorrect latching means less milk gets through, your supply dwindles in response, and baby wants to nurse around-the-clock in desperation!

- **More is more.** Try increasing feeds – the more you nurse, the more milk you make. It's that simple really. Crank up your sessions to at least every one to two hours daily and aim for three-hourly feeds at night.

- **Empty both breasts.** Even swap sides during a feed (especially if baby is falling asleep or getting distracted).

- **Ditch the dummy.** Allowing her to satisfy her suckling needs at the breast automatically makes more milk.

- **Take a break.** Clearing the decks for a bit and simply lounging about—or in bed—with baby at the breast is a fabulous way to de-stress and re-ignite milk production.

- **The world can wait.** Sleep when baby sleeps, drink to thirst, eat a lot and look after yourself.

- **Don't give water, formula or solids under six months.** If baby is older, you could increase milk and decrease solids for a while.

- **Pumping between feeds steps up milk production.** To make sure you're squeezing out the greatest amount of milk possible, continue pumping for at least five minutes after the last few drips.

"I thought my milk had dried up at six weeks. Nobody had told me that the milk storage process changes around then, and your breasts stop feeling full. If a friend hadn't told me just in time I would have continued with switching her to formula! Instead I fed for a full two years with no problem – and no bottles."

Nicole, 32, mum to Karly, 3.

Golly! A galactagogue!

When a friend first mentioned that I should try one of these, I didn't know what she on about. After purchasing one (I'm keeping you in suspense) my supply sky-rocketed and I burst forth in a shower of milky sparks. Took a half-dose from then on. Galactagogues are substances thought to increase milk supply. You'll find all sorts at your local pharmacy or health shop and everyone has opinions on which are best. Only a test run will reveal which one's for you. The most common are:

- Alfalfa (I used this – delicious, raspberry-flavoured, powerful and moreish).
- Blessed thistle.
- Fenugreek.

It's best to first try to increase your milk supply using the hints above or chat to a lactation consultant or La Leche League before going the medicinal route – holistic or otherwise. Chances are you don't have a low supply.

If you absolutely do (or want to take something just to be sure) then there's also prescription medication available from your doctor. Also, don't take anything at all without your doctor or pharmacist's say so! I'd rest up and try out these tips first. My supply went completely overboard thanks to my galactagogue and I ended up with engorged breasts. Can't win, eh?!

Mammary myths exposed

It's nobody's fault that antiquated, ignorant breastfeeding information is still being fed to new mums like so much chocolate gateau. The attitude 'if it ain't broke, why fix it?' is understandable, considering that the human race still survives the onslaught of shortened nursing relationships and mass marketing of formula. But merely surviving isn't enough – living healthily and as nature intended is the grand prize to aim for, not so?

With that in mind, let's lay some lactation cards on the table and put to rest, once and for all, a couple of ridiculous myths about breastfeeding:

- **My milk is weak!** This is so much codswallop. Breasts are designed for making milk and even malnourished women are able to feed their babies – the body simply draws sufficient nutrients from the mother's body. Put your mind at ease by talking to a trained lactation consultant if necessary, but don't allow general medical professionals to bully you into switching to formula.

- **I don't have enough!** Close to 100 per cent of women are able to breastfeed. Only the tiniest percentage is unable to for very specific medical reasons. With solid nutritional advice (a normal diet and plenty of fluids), adequate rest, assistance with correct latching and demand feeding, you can be sure that you have enough milk.

- **Time to give up!** She's teething. What nonsense! If baby bites (which is rare), say "no" in a stern voice and refuse to nurse for a few minutes. She'll usually lead up to the bite anyway, so you'll know when your cherubic cobra is about to strike. The "no" and removal of nipple usually does the trick though.

- **Feeding routines are fab.** For mum initially, perhaps, but they don't work. Your body's milk supply and demand system needs you to feed on cue. It won't be long before she finds her own routine and you'll have a break for hours at a time.

- **Bed-feeding is spoiling her.** Such rot. Affection, bonding and the relaxed nature of nursing in the family bed is one of the best ways to bring up a healthy baby. You'll also sleep longer and better.

- **She must have both breasts.** Sure, it's better to empty both – but some babies prefer one and will go for it more frequently and enthusiastically. It is more than possible to feed a baby with only one breast – you will simply make more milk and she'll feed more frequently to compensate.

I am beautiful as I am.
I am the shape that
was gifted. My breasts
are no longer perky
and upright like when
I was a teenager.
My hips are wider
than that of a fashion
model's. For this I am
glad, for these are the
signs of a life lived.

Cindy Olsen

Boobs, bottles, bosses & such

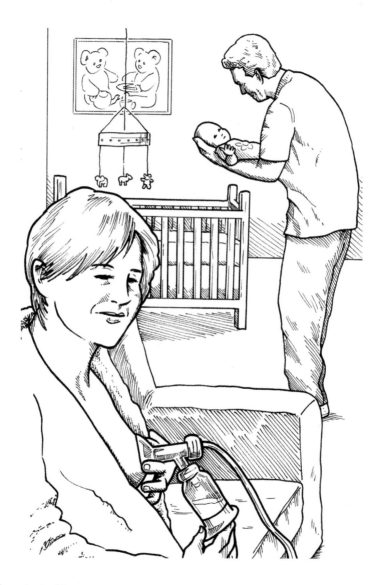

chapter 10
Boobs, bottles, bosses & such

End of an era

At some point in your breastfeeding relationship, things change. Perhaps you're going back to work; perchance baby has to be hospitalised for some reason, or she's ready to start solids. You may even just want a weekend away! All these factors greatly influence how—or if—you're going to continue nursing.

For many mums, the slightest development signals the end of milk-making. But before you take that lactation leap, consider the fact that breastfeeding is still possible (and even fun!) under virtually any circumstance.

> ### Quick tip
>
> **THE WORKING MUM**
> You can still breastfeed exclusively if you plan ahead. Experts say that mums can go back to work half-days without leaving bottles of expressed milk or formula, as long as your baby is at least five months old. When baby is closer to a year—from about 10 months—you can feed mornings and evenings only, meaning a full-time job is possible.

Express yourself

For whatever reason, you might find yourself bending over a bottle late at night, boobs dangling, milking yourself like the proverbial cow. Alternatively, you'll buy a fancy, battery-operated, hospital-grade pump and hook yourself up, avoiding smirks and stifled laughs from your partner. Expressing milk is often a necessity and always rather comical. So what makes mums express?

- You need to be away from baby and won't be able to feed her at the breast.
- You're taking medication and need to 'pump and dump' in order to keep your supply going until you can nurse her again.
- You're trying to build up your supply.
- You'd like a darn break! Let your partner give her a bottle of mum's milk for a change, I hear you say.

Pump it up!

We're spoiled for choice these days, with several handy gadgets on the market designed to make removing milk that much easier and trouble-free. The cheaper ones are manually operated (I couldn't get to grips with these) while more expensive ones are usually electric (battery or mains) for personal home use. I found that these removed milk fast and furiously. For interest's sake, the hospital-grade pumps for multiple users are quite phenomenal – I used one while in hospital for a gall bladder removal. Samara was just eight months old and I was anxious to keep up my supply. I watched in awe as my breasts spewed out floods of milk in minutes. Still, at home, I hand-expressed when necessary. You'll find your own 'zone' too.